B53 023 763 6

KT-494-608

Strength and Power Training For Martial Arts

Strength and Power Training For Martial Arts

by
Martina Sprague

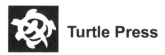 Turtle Press   Hartford

STRENGTH AND POWER TRAINING FOR MARTIAL ARTS

Copyright © 2005 Martina Sprague. All rights reserved. Printed in the United States of America. No part of this book may be reproduced without written permission except in the case of brief quotations embodied in articles or reviews. For information, address Turtle Press, PO Box 290206,Wethersfield CT 06129-0206.

To contact the author or to order additional copies of this book:
  Turtle Press
  P.O. Box 290206
  Wethersfield, CT 06129-0206
  1-880-77-TURTL

ISBN 1-880336-87-1
LCCN   2005006278
Printed in the United States of America

10 9 8 7 6 5 4 3

Library of Congress Cataloguing in Publication Data
Sprague, Martina.
 Strength and power training for martial arts / by Martina Sprague.-- 1st ed.
    p. cm.
  ISBN 1-880336-87-1
 1. Martial arts--Training. I. Title.
  GV1102.7.T7S67 2005
  613.7'148--dc22
                    2005006278

ROTHERHAM LIBRARY SERVICE	
B53023763	
Bertrams	11/07/2012
AN	£16.95
DIN	613.7148

To Margareta Westin, my lifelong friend.

Acknowledgements:

My sincere thanks go to Scott, Nicholas, and Parker Fluehe, and to Alan Lamm for posing for the photographs.

I would also like to express my appreciation to Tony Martinez, Sr. and to Gold's Gym in West Valley, Utah for granting me permission to photograph on-site.

And, as always, many thanks to my fantastic publisher, Turtle Press.

Contents

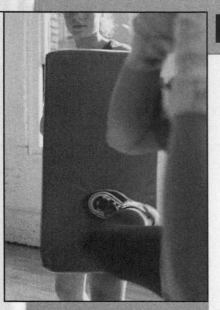

Introduction

In this section:

- **Myths & Facts**

- **Quick Reference to Strength Training Concepts**

- **Introduction**

Fact, Fiction, and Half-Truths

Strength training is a subject of continuous exploration and scientific findings. New discoveries are made and old beliefs discarded. While some of the common strength training "myths" have some validity, it is important to understand where they stemmed from and why you should take them with a grain of salt. I also warn against using absolutes, such as *"always* do this" or *"never* do that." For example, a few common absolutes in strength training are: *Never* do full situps, straight leg situps, or clasp your hands behind your neck, *always* train the larger muscle groups prior to training the smaller muscle groups, *always* exhale on the positive phase and inhale on the negative phase of a lift, *always* see a physician before starting a new exercise program.

The key to success is education. With education comes a greater understanding of the particular body you possess, which leads to the ability to tweak these absolutes to your advantage. In other words, when you come to know your own body and capabilities, you can break the rules. For example, I have found that for me (although not necessarily for you) full situps and straight leg situps are good ab exercises. And the reason you shouldn't clasp your hands behind your neck is to avoid pulling against your neck when it is really the abs you are working. But if you don't pull against your neck . . . well, you get my drift. Furthermore, sometimes circumstances are such that it might benefit you more to train the smaller muscle groups prior to training the larger muscle groups. And as far as breathing goes, I sometimes do very quick "sprint" repetitions that require a different breathing pattern, for example, exhaling on every other lift instead of on every lift, or even holding my breath for short durations of time.

On the subject of seeing a physician before starting a new exercise program, I think it is a good idea, although the point is that every person must know for him or herself what is appropriate, based on his or her education and background. For example, if you have been exercising all of your life, chances are you probably have a pretty good idea of what you are capable of, more so than any physician can tell you. On the other hand, if you are older and just starting out, you might (but not necessarily) have different needs. My opinion is therefore that some of these absolutes don't benefit you and have been overused primarily to guard against lawsuits should something go wrong. But as the owner of your body, you alone carry the responsibility to research your needs, to take appropriate safety precautions, and to do what is right for you. Before you dive into the material presented in this book, go ahead and explore, research, and think about the following facts, fictions, and half-truths.

Myth: It is all in the technique, and you don't need strength to be a successful martial artist.

Fact: Technique is important, and technique along with intelligence and courage can help a smaller or weaker person defeat a larger adversary. However, strength *does* matter. Strength increases your confidence, helps you achieve your objectives with greater ease, and raises your pain threshold, allowing you to endure greater physical punishment.

Myth: Lifting weights will improve your martial arts skills.

Fact: Weight training will make you stronger; skills training will improve your martial arts skills. However, a stronger athlete has the potential to be a better athlete. A strong martial artist can hit harder, throw higher and more powerful kicks, endure more pain, outrun an assailant, or intimidate a group of bullies.

Myth: Weight training makes you "muscle-bound" and reduces flexibility, and is therefore detrimental to the martial artist.

Fact: Weight training does not reduce flexibility. In fact, lifting weights through a limb's entire range of motion, or doing negatives that allow the muscle to lengthen, is likely to increase flexibility. Also, when your muscles are warm after you have completed the exercise, you can stretch the muscles easier.

Myth: Weight training will make you slow.

Fact: Stronger muscles can make you faster and more explosive, and stronger muscles will definitely not make you lose speed in your martial arts techniques.

Myth: Carrying dumbbells or ankle weights when you walk or run helps improve muscular strength.

Fact: Dumbbells or ankle weights are not heavy enough to help build muscular strength. They also slow you down, so you

might not benefit as much in cardiovascular terms. In addition, they change your timing, for example, when throwing a punch or kick, and could therefore be detrimental to your sport.

Myth: Aerobic fitness is more important than muscular strength.

Fact: Aerobic fitness is important. What most people don't know is that one of the most efficient ways to build aerobic fitness is through high intensity resistance training (weight lifting), and not through elliptical trainers or aerobic classes. Weight lifting saves time and allows you to catch "two flies with one swat" (and these are bigger flies than what you'll catch by prioritizing aerobics).

Myth: Sweating while exercising means you are unfit or overweight.

Fact: Sweating is the body's way of cooling itself, and sweating a lot means that you have an efficient cooling system. However, cranking up the temperature, wearing too much clothing, or wearing an airtight suit in order to induce sweating can be detrimental and can even cause death through heatstroke in rare instances. Sweat to keep cool, not to "sweat out the extra weight." It won't happen.

Myth: Muscles turn to fat when you stop exercising.

Fact: Muscles and fat are different tissues and one tissue does not become another. Muscles don't turn to fat; you get fat as a result of eating more than what you use up. When you stop exercising, muscles atrophy, and if you don't also reduce the amount of calories you eat, you will pack on the fat pounds.

Myth: Low intensity exercise is a greater "fat burner" than high intensity exercise, and therefore contributes to greater weight loss.

Fact: Carbohydrates are a more efficient source of energy than is fat. At low intensity exercise, the body doesn't need to be efficient, so it uses fat instead of carbohydrates. But the idea that low intensity exercise is a great fat burner is a misconception that doesn't hold up mathematically, because when you engage in high intensity training, you use up a greater percentage of calories in the same amount of time, so high intensity training is, in fact, a greater "fat burner" than low intensity training.

Myth: Muscles that don't show are not strong.

Fact: Muscles only show if you have a lean body. Excess fat will cover up the muscles and is especially prevalent around the midsection on most people. But muscles that don't show can be just as strong as muscles that do show. Yes, you can be both strong and fat. In fact, being too lean or over-obsessing about your diet can be detrimental to your health. Work to improve strength, not looks.

Myth: When you have reached 40, you will experience little benefit from strength training.

Fact: Older men and women achieve favorable benefits from strength training. The fact that older people often have less strength than younger people is due to a decrease in muscle mass, which is further due to the fact that many people, as they age (usually around the age of 40-50), become less active. Older people need to stay active and continue strength training in order to keep their muscle mass. Exercise can help delay the loss of lean tissue, such as muscle, for decades in the older population. Therefore, old does not automatically equate to weak. "A group from a residential home for elderly in Boston aged between 86 and 96 was put on a six-week strength program. Exercises were restricted to the thigh muscles (quadriceps) and the program consisted solely of strength training, ie no walking exercises, stretching or gymnastics. The average increase in strength was 174%; CT scans measured a 9% increase in muscle tissue. Walking speeds increased by 48%." (www.kieser-training.com)

Myth: It is dangerous to start lifting weights when you are older, if you are not already in good shape.

Fact: It is never too late to start strength training, but you should understand the demands you place on your body and use a progressive program. Building a strong body takes time, both for youngsters and seniors. Don't expect to accomplish your goal in one day.

Myth: If you can't afford a gym membership, you can't gain maximum benefit from a strength-training program.

Fact: Bodyweight exercises, or exercises that rely on the movement of your body (for example, pushups, pull-ups, situps, squats, and lunges) as opposed to the movement of an external weight, are some of the most effective exercises for improving sport specific strength, and can be done at increased resistance by working on an incline or by using only one arm or leg.

Myth: The concentric phase of a lift is more important than the eccentric phase.

Fact: The concentric or positive phase is where you lift the weight; the eccentric or negative phase is where you lower the weight. Both involve muscular contraction. As long as you don't rely on gravity to do the work for you, in some instances the eccentric phase can be even more beneficial than the concentric phase, helping you push past your previous threshold.

Myth: Women don't have the genetic makeup to benefit from strength training.

Fact: Women's muscle fibers are identical to men's muscle fibers, and women can (and should) engage in identical strength-training programs. Women are often smaller than men and don't have the same testosterone levels, but this is not an excuse for making strength training gender specific.

Myth: Strength training for women could be detrimental, because women might develop muscles that are unsightly and make them look unfeminine.

Fact: This is not possible, because women don't have the testosterone required to build huge and unsightly muscles. If you see a women with very well defined muscles, it is likely that she has been on a strict diet that has cut all the subcutaneous fat (just below the skin's surface), so the muscles show better. You might see this in competitive female bodybuilders, but not in other athletes that are using strength training as a supplement to their sport (we are going by the assumption that no anabolic steroids were used). Besides, it takes a lot of work for both men and women to grow muscles of considerable size. If only we were so lucky that we had to fear "bulking up."

Myth: Women are more flexible than men.

Fact: Keep in mind that women are often smaller than men, and a smaller person has a shorter distance to reach in order to touch his or her toes. If the legs are shorter, the groin will be closer to the ground when attempting the splits. A smaller person might therefore appear more flexible, but this is a visual illusion. When doing the splits, it is the angle between the legs that determines flexibility, not how close the groin is to the ground.

Myth: Weight lifting is dangerous for your joints.

Fact: Any improper lift, with or without weights, can injure your joints, especially your back. Exercises, such as squats, that are generally considered dangerous for the knees, will not hurt healthy joints if you use proper technique. If you have a prior injury, you may need to alter or avoid certain exercises.

Myth: Machine weight training is safer than free weight training.

Fact: Both machine and free weight training are very safe when performed correctly, and have fewer injuries than most other sports. When lifting heavy free weights, you might need a spotter to assist you, but it is not the free weight movement in itself that increases the risk of injury.

Myth: You shouldn't train while you are injured.

Fact: Generally, it is a good idea to continue training in at least some form or way while recovering from an injury. Continuing training will prevent muscle atrophy. However, it is important not to aggravate the injured body part. Some injuries might require complete rest.

Myth: The more, the better.

Fact: You need adequate rest to avoid over-training and allow your muscles to become stronger. 48 hours is recommended between training sessions. Shorter and well-planned workouts are recommended over long hours at the gym.

Myth: No pain, no gain.

Fact: Well, it depends on what type of pain you are referring to. You can't expect to reach great results if you don't put in your time. Thus, a 5-minute a day workout program is not going to cut it, nor is lifting 5-pound dumbbells 20 times. When you get fatigued, it will hurt. So, yes there is going to be pain if you want gain. However, the pain that is unwelcome is the pain that results from overuse injuries or incorrect lifting techniques.

Quick Reference to Strength Training Concepts

The following strength training concepts will help you optimize your lifting technique and performance, so that you can reach your goal with the least amount of wasted effort. Develop a good understanding of the concepts, and keep them in mind whenever you go to the gym to train. The concepts are listed in alphabetical order. For a more complete discussion, please refer to Chapter 5 on Understanding the Concepts.

Acceleration

Accelerate the weight briefly and quickly, not evenly throughout the lift. Brief maximal efforts improve force development and ability to accelerate heavy loads. The move must be controlled. Do not rely on momentum.

Breathing

Exhale on the positive (concentric) phase, and inhale on the negative (eccentric) phase of the lift. Correct breathing technique helps you focus your strength and maximize your workout.

Flexibility

Improve flexibility by working your muscles through full range of motion. Avoid cheating. Do not do partial lifts.

Goal Oriented Training

Know your reasons for training; know what you are trying to achieve. Being goal oriented helps you accomplish more per training session.

Intensity

Use heavy weights and few repetitions as opposed to lighter weights and more repetitions. In addition to genetics, the intensity of your workout (how heavy loads you use) is the most important factor determining growth of muscular strength.

Machines or Free Weights

Be more concerned with intensity of training than with equipment used. Both machines and free weights are good, as long as you use heavy enough loads. If you can do more than 8 repetitions, increase the load.

Mechanics and Momentum

Use proper lifting technique before increasing the resistance. Improper mechanics, such as the use of momentum, are not a true measure of your strength and can cause injuries. Pausing briefly, 2-3 seconds, at full range involves a slight isometric contraction, helps eliminate momentum, and allows you to build strength in your weakest link.

Midsection

Prioritize training the midsection. The midsection is the connective link between the lower and upper body and is used in virtually every move you make. If training the midsection seems unimportant, do your abdominal work prior to all other training in order to ensure that it gets done.

Multiple Muscle Groups

Use exercises that target multiple muscle groups at a time; for example, lunges and squats (quadriceps, hamstrings, glutes, calves). These are more beneficial and time-economical than exercises that isolate the muscle groups; for example, leg extensions (quadriceps) and hamstring curls (hamstrings).

Muscle Mass and Strength

Maximize strength by lifting heavy weights (90% of your 1-rep maximum), doing a low number of repetitions (3-8), and using long rest periods between sets (2-4 minutes). Significant hypertrophy (growth of muscle) is primarily based on genetic inheritance, and does not necessarily communicate your functional muscular strength.

Muscular Endurance

Perform exercises with no or minimal rest between muscle group workouts when training for muscular endurance. Do a greater number of repetitions per set: 1-2 sets, 12-20 reps are recommended. If you are unable to do 12 reps, decrease the load.

If you can do more than 20 reps, increase the load. Rest no more than 1 minute between exercises.

Muscular Failure

Muscular failure means that you are unable to do another rep. You can realize results without training to muscular failure; however, training to failure every so often might serve as a gauge to let you know what you are capable of.

Muscular Strength

Perform exercises with longer rest periods between muscle group workouts when training for muscular strength. Do a lower number of repetitions per set: 2-3 sets, 6-10 reps are recommended. If you can do more than 10 reps, increase the load. Rest for 2-4 minutes between exercises.

Negatives

Take advantage of negative lifts. Strength training techniques are divided into positive (concentric) and negative (eccentric) moves. The positive move is when you lift the weight, and the negative move is when you lower the weight. When you have reached muscular failure on the positive move, you can usually do a couple of negative repetitions before your muscles are exhausted.

Opposing Muscle Groups

Train opposing muscle groups. Failing to do so results in muscle imbalance and can cause muscle pulls or strains of the weaker muscle. For example, if you train the quadriceps, you must also train the hamstrings. If you train the biceps, you must also train the triceps. If you train the chest, you must also train the back.

Over-Training

Beware of the negative effects of over-training. If you train your body beyond its capability to recover, you will experience the symptoms of over-training. These include muscle soreness, general lack of energy, lethargy or a burned out feeling. Lack of proper rest and recovery has an adverse effect on your physical and mental well-being.

Progressive Overload

Overload your muscles by setting a progressive schedule. In order to realize muscular *strength* gains, stress your muscles against greater loads. In order to realize muscular *endurance* gains, work your muscles for longer periods of time. As you adapt to the training and your regimen is getting easier, increase the load to make it more difficult.

Range of Motion

Use full range of motion when lifting weights. Using partial range of motion might allow you to do more repetitions, but you won't achieve the maximum strength benefit. It is better to do fewer repetitions with good form and full range of motion.

Recovery Time

Rest after a strenuous workout. Your body needs time to recover, about 48 hours is recommended. Sometimes you need time to recover from an injury or to get over burnout.

Repeated Submaximal Efforts

Do several repetitions using slightly less than maximum intensity to develop basic strength, basic muscle mass, muscular endurance, and stamina.

Specificity

Improve your strength, not your martial arts skills, through the use of strength training. In order to determine whether a strength training exercise is skill specific, it must pass four tests: muscle specificity, movement specificity, speed specificity, and resistance specificity. Few (if any) strength exercises pass this test.

Sport Specific Exercises

Choose exercises that are specific to the type of strength you need the most; for example, upper body strength, lower body strength, explosive strength, muscular endurance strength, gripping strength, and cardiovascular strength. Note that muscular endurance and cardiovascular endurance are not the same. Muscular endurance refers to the major muscles in your body, and cardiovascular endurance refers exclusively to the capacity of your heart.

Uneven and Unstable Surfaces

Train on uneven or unstable surfaces, such as a slope or a stability ball, to increase the difficulty of an exercise. Training on uneven or unstable surfaces requires a greater muscular effort in order to keep your balance, and therefore helps you achieve greater strength gains. Do not train on uneven or unstable surfaces until you can do the exercise with good form on a stable surface.

Tensing

Tense your muscles prior to doing a strength training exercise, such as a pushup. Tensing makes the exercise seem easier than if you start with your muscles relaxed, and allows you to increase the load.

Variation

Vary the exercises used or the frequency and length of training sessions to avoid falling into a rut that stops challenging muscular growth. Failing to vary your routines will make your body adapt, and muscular strength building will cease.

Introduction

Why strength-train? Because the secret to great martial arts performance does not lie in technique alone, but also in how well you can manipulate your body against a variety of forces. These include your own weight, your opponent's weight, and inertia for quick changes in speed and direction. Many sports make an effort to match you as closely as possible to your competitors. For example, you will be grouped according to your gender, age, weight, height, and skill level or number of years in the sport. You will be weighed, sometimes measured, and asked to disclose your rank or competition record. This is done in an effort to level the playing field. But have you ever heard of a martial arts competition that required you to take a strength test prior to entering?

The ability to exert your strength properly and at the right moment gives you a competitive edge over your opponent. When you are physically strong, your acceleration, body balance, recovery, and reaction time improve and make you an overall more efficient fighter. This is true whether you compete in free sparring, techniques, forms, or breaking. Your strength may be of even greater importance in situations that do not make allowances for differences in gender, age, weight, height, or skill level and background; for example, when you are faced with a real adversary on the street. Superior strength and conditioning might allow you to outrun an attacker, ward off an assault, physically injure an assailant, and recover from sustained injuries quicker. Superior strength and conditioning establish your reputation as a formidable opponent that is not to be messed with, in or out of the ring or competition arena. Having a strong and well-conditioned body also sharpens your mental edge. When you know that you can take your opponent the distance, your confidence grows, and with it your motivation and warrior spirit, both of which are important to outdo your competition.

A good general fitness base is a must to ensure that your body is ready to participate in athletic performance at the spur of the moment, and not just "in season." Part of this book is devoted to educating you on the importance of strength training and fitness, and to give you knowledge of different strength training methods. Once you have achieved a general fitness base, you will feel more inclined to put your plans into practice. This is because you have readied your body for exercise and you no longer need to question the validity of the principles. The rest of the book is devoted to giving you the ability to design a martial art specific strength and conditioning program. The general fitness principles are valid for all people, but the martial art specific programs are based on the art you practice and on your personal physical and mental characteristics.

In order to make good use of such a program, you need to educate yourself on several factors affecting athletic performance. These factors must then be interrelated and work together in order to maximize the gain for the effort:

1. **Exercise physiology and human anatomy**, or the study of inherited genetic factors such as muscle build, bone structure and body functions, and how to design exercises that target specific muscle groups

2. **Biomechanics**, or the study of the principles of movement in a human being in relation to martial arts and strength training

3. **Physics**, or the study of natural laws of motion that help or hinder performance

4. **Psychology**, or how to gain a

mental edge, including how to approach your training or an upcoming competition

5. **Outside factors,** such as your ability to understand and adapt to variations in your opponent's build or in the environment

When you have achieved the educational background and understand the science of strength training, your next step is to think through your specific needs and physical qualities, and then tweak your training program in such a way that you can derive the most benefit from it. To start, you may want to look at what can be significantly improved through training. Although you can improve in most areas, such as strength, power, and speed, some of our physical traits are inherited and unchangeable. Everybody does not have the same capacity to improve to the same degree. This makes certain types of training more beneficial to some people than to others. For example, physical build, flexibility, and capacity to develop strength and explosiveness differ between individuals. A good understanding of your genetic capacity helps you tailor a program so that you can reap the greatest benefits in practical terms.

In order to create a useful program, we must toss out factors that are based purely on opinion. Although personal experience can be valuable and often helps drive home a point, it should not be assumed that what worked for me will also work for you, or vice versa. A good program is based on defining how and why a move, technique, or routine works and finding a way to incorporate it into your training. Start by identifying and focusing on your objective: to become a better, stronger, faster martial artist (not to become a better or stronger power lifter, or to become a more physically attractive person). Although power lifting is impressive and physical attraction is a bonus, they should not be your primary

focus. Your goal is to develop the physique and stamina that enable you to do what needs to be done when engaged in your particular style of martial art. Don't lose sight of your goal.

Next, learn the different types of exercises that will build your strength. Also think about the moves and techniques your martial art requires, and how a specific type of strength is to be used in your art. For example, does the strength exercise help you throw a more powerful punch or a higher kick? Does the strength exercise give you the stamina you need to dominate your opponent and back him into the ropes? No strength training technique is an island. Every lift, twist, push, pull, drive, or shove has a greater purpose.

Your strength-training program must also be designed so that you can stick with it for the long haul; the methods must be time-economical and interesting. Most of us have other obligations outside of our martial arts training, so a program that requires five hours a day is impractical. In order to maintain motivation, the goals you set must be achievable within the limits of your schedule, or they are of little value.

With the exception of the chapter on women's strength training, which specifically targets those women who still doubt the benefits of developing strong and not just toned muscles, all parts of this book apply equally to men and women. The strength and fitness education you gather from this book, along with the many sample exercises, will help you establish the kind of training program that benefits you the most. In the end, you alone are responsible for maintaining your health and fitness. In order to win, you must prepare to win. Your success depends on a well-constructed program along with commitment and passion.

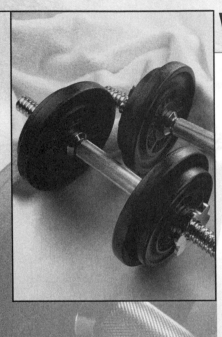

What is Strength?

In this section:

- Factors affecting strength

- Classifying your martial arts

- What requires strength?

- General strength base

- Developing impressive strength

- Your training program

- Summing it up

What is Strength?

I am sure you can remember a time on the street, in the gym, or in the martial arts training hall when another person's physique made you turn around and think, "If only I had a build like yours." An impressive body gives you physical and psychological advantages over an opponent. Just the fact that you turned and looked at another person is an indication that his or her build had an effect on you. We normally relate being muscular to being strong, healthy, and capable, all of which are qualities we, as martial artist, desire. As far as strength goes, there is physical strength, mental strength, and relative strength, or the kind of strength that changes depending on the situation and circumstances. The primary focus of this book is physical strength. But even physical strength needs to be further defined in order to have meaning.

How do we measure physical strength? Is it measured by your Arnold Schwarzenegger look? How long you can last in a sparring match? Your 1-repetition maximum in a given exercise, such as the bench press? How fast you can run a mile? How many pushups, pull-ups, dips, and squats you can do? These types of definitions are not useful, because you are not defining what is important. That is, unless you are particularly training to win a 1-mile race or to excel at a pushup contest. But if you are training for the martial arts, or more specifically for Kenpo karate, Tae-Kwon-Do, Jijutsu, or even more specifically to win the next tournament in forms or sparring, you must define your strength goals in more definite terms.

When getting started in a strength-training program for the martial arts, it is not muscle toning or weight loss you are aiming for, nor is it the Arnold Schwarzenegger look. Physical strength involves more than how many pounds you can lift. Look at physical strength:

• **In Relation to Your Opponent.** If you are physically stronger than your opponent, you can dominate him or her. Since this is relative strength, it changes depending on whom you are fighting.

• **In Relation to Your Own Bodyweight.** Since the martial arts are traditionally focused around empty-hand combat where you generally don't have a strength equalizer such as a knife or a handgun, how successful you are depends on your ability to move and use the natural weapons of your body. The traditional karate weapons, such as the sword, staff, or nunchaku also require considerable strength to wield with explosive power.

Regardless of how you define it, physical strength is an important quality because it gives you power, speed, explosiveness, endurance, and a fierce appearance, all of which are winning attributes in the fighting arts.

Factors affecting strength

How strong you are depends on the circumstances under which you fight:

• **Your clothing** affects your strength. Your clothing might be cumbersome, restrict your mobility, or drain strength from you by keeping your body from cooling itself effectively.

• **The temperature**, both hot and cold, affects your strength. Heat can make you feel drained and dehydrated, and cold can make you feel stiff and slow.

• **The terrain** affects your strength. Fighting on uneven, unstable, or slick surfaces forces you to tense or use different muscles than fighting on flat surfaces with good traction.

• **An injury**, even a relatively minor one such as a pulled muscle, affects your strength and may place more stress on other body parts to help protect the one that is injured.

Sometimes your strength is related to how well you utilize your expertise in technique and strategy. Other factors that affect your strength include your preparation, your health on the particular day you need to use your strength, whether you are hungry, thirsty, or tired, mental distractions and baggage you might be carrying, your level of confidence, and your general energy level, which is further affected by your previous experiences or factors that might have fatigued you.

Classifying your martial art

Are the martial arts endurance or power sports? Are muscular strength, muscular endurance, and power the same things?

• **Muscular strength** is your ability to lift a heavy weight once.

• **Muscular endurance** is your ability to last through a longer period of physical exertion, or to lift a weight several times in succession.

• **Power** is your ability to use your strength in a sudden, explosive move.

Endurance sports are typically defined as sports that require you to maintain your speed for a long duration of time, such as distance running or swimming. Power sports are typically defined as sports that require quick acceleration, deceleration, changes in direction, or explosive jumping, such as sprinting or gymnastics. How would you classify your martial art? Does the style you study impact the classification, or are all arts the same? If you classify your art primarily as a power art, can you still be successful if you treat it as an endurance art?

Just as one approach to strategy doesn't work for all fighters, one approach to strength training doesn't work for all fighters. But generally, the martial arts are classified as power sports, and more emphasis should be placed on developing strength and power rather than endurance. I am not suggesting that you ignore endurance, but your main focus should not be on running 10 miles a day.

What requires strength?

Some people seem naturally gifted when it comes to strength. They have low body fat and a muscular or impressive upper body. To a degree it is true that some people are born with "better" genes for developing an impressive physique. If you aren't one of them, you might shrug and ask, "What's the use?" But rather than thinking in terms of how you look, define what strength means to you. What exactly do you need in order to succeed in your martial art? This includes more than a list of the techniques you need to master. For example, you must determine the frequency and level at which these techniques are to be performed. Do you need to be strong enough to participate in martial arts class three days a week? Compete twice a month?

The type of strength required to climb a rope to escape an adversary on the street differs from the type of strength needed to compete in next month's point sparring tournament. One type of strength is not necessarily better than another, but you should know how the type of strength you are seeking relates to your martial art.

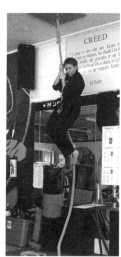

Attending morning classes might require a different type of strength than attending evening classes when you have already completed a full day's work. Attending classes as a family activity requires a different type of strength than competing at a vigorous level. Note that I'm not saying that the martial arts as a family activity require less impressive strength; what I'm saying is that your strength requirements relate to what you wish to achieve. The point is that strength is not black and white; it is not extreme. There are many levels of strength. To say that you are either strong or not has no meaning, unless you also relate it to what you wish to achieve.

Strength is a measure of your ability to set yourself in motion against a counterweight or resistance, and in some cases to maintain motion for extended periods of time. How well you perform in the martial arts is a result of how efficiently you use your body. This includes:

- Forward, reverse and side-to-side movement

- Getting down on the ground and getting up from the ground

- Pulling, pushing and twisting

- Striking, kicking, blocking and grabbing

- Jumping

Most of your martial arts techniques involve speed, explosiveness, balance, coordination, and flexibility, all of which are built on strength and the ability to transfer power from the lower body to the upper body, or vice versa. Power, for example, involves your ability to contract your muscles and explode in a coordinated effort at the right moment. Punching involves the transfer of power from your legs to your body and arms. Kicking involves balance and the transfer of power from your body, or from one leg to the other. Your upper and lower body must be coordinated for quick, balanced, and powerful motion. If your arms are faster than your legs, you can't propel yourself forward with efficiency, or you risk injury or balance loss by over-extending your center of gravity. There are also twisting motions required when throwing strikes or pushing against your opponent. These require strength in the midsection as well as in the legs. Important skills include the ability to press forward when throwing a strike or kick, or to press against and manipulate the weight of your opponent's body. You need strength for:

Balance

When you are fighting on uneven surfaces, there is more muscular tension on one leg or one side of your body than on the other. The same is true when fighting on unstable surfaces. For us who practice only in the martial arts training hall, uneven or unstable surfaces might not be an issue, but consider what happens if you need to use your skill for real; for example, on the rolling deck of a ship, where you need to adjust to the sudden forces of the sea.

Striking and Driving

Most martial arts use a combination of quick, snappy techniques such as a front snap kick, and techniques that require a longer time commitment such as wrestling your opponent to the ground. Your weight will always work to your advantage when utilizing striking and driving techniques. The same is true for muscular strength. A strong fighter can drive farther before his muscles fail him. This type of fighter can therefore be more successful in a fight that does not rely solely on light or no contact sparring. But even in light or no contact martial arts, muscular strength is required for deep stances, lengthy demonstrations, and when wielding a weapon.

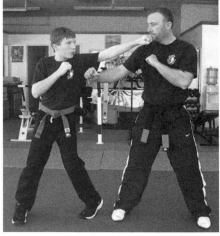

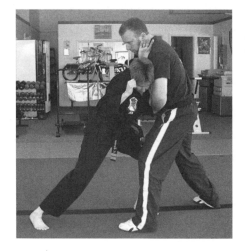

Muscular strength and good mechanics can give a smaller person the advantage when striking (above) and driving (left).

Wielding Weapons

Working with the traditional martial arts weapons, such as the sword, stick, staff, or nunchaku requires strength. Success with such weapons depends on your ability to wield them with speed, power, and determination. The longer and heavier the weapon, the more strength is required to manipulate it. Without adequate strength, you are likely to telegraph your moves, use sloppy swings, strike without speed, or fail to withdraw the weapon in preparation for a new attack. You need strength in your upper body, lower body, and midsection to wield a traditional weapon successfully.

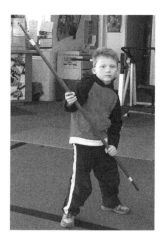

The longer and heavier the weapon, the more strength is required to wield it with speed and power.

Jumping

If you are involved in competitions requiring aerial maneuvers, you must know how to jump and spin while maintaining balance. High jumps require leg strength and explosiveness. Your upper body contributes with movement and balance and helps you achieve height in the jump.

A jump kick therefore requires a combination of upper and lower body strength.

Developing a general strength base

If you have not participated in a strength-training program for some time, you must build your strength gradually to avoid injuries. You must develop a general strength and fitness base before you can benefit from sport specific training. A general fitness base is required for any sport, and is comprised of muscular strength and endurance, cardiovascular fitness, and flexibility. Without this base, it is difficult to establish a competitive edge in your particular type of sport. See Chapter 8 on Building Your Strength Base, and move forward within the following guidelines:

• **Develop general aerobic fitness** and strength endurance in your lower body, upper body, and midsection.

• **Develop good mobility** and flexibility in your joints.

• **Develop muscular endurance**. Strength is not absolute. In other words, it is not only about how heavy a weight you can lift once at a specific moment, but also about for how long you can sustain a muscular effort.

• **Develop anaerobic strength**, which allows you to exert maximum strength in repeated spurts.

Once you start developing a general fitness base, you will begin seeing improvements within a few weeks in your ability to perform in your art. You will notice greater endurance and less fatigue. This is because you are training your body to accept the higher demands placed upon it, and it is adapting and getting stronger and more energetic. As you lay this foundation, you will start gaining confidence in your abilities. General athletic fitness gives you the base you need to prevent injuries and be reasonably ready to participate in your sport at the spur of the moment.

Developing impressive strength

The most effective way to increase strength is by increasing muscle mass. The most effective way to increase muscle mass is through weight or resistance training involving heavy loads. Hypertrophy, or the growth of muscles, occurs when the intensity of the workload is increased. The intensity can be thought of as the resistance. A high load and few repetitions result in more muscular growth than a light load and many repetitions. When strength is increased so are speed and power, because speed and power depend on muscle contraction.

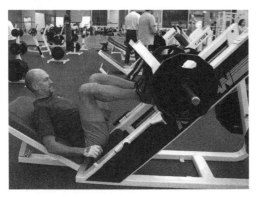

Working with weights is more effective for the purpose of increasing muscle mass, than are aerobic devices.

Strength can be broken down into muscular strength (how much you can lift), muscular endurance (how long you can keep going against a specific resistance), and explosive strength (how quickly you can set your body in motion and exert your strength for a specific purpose). For example:

- Muscular strength = one-armed pushups.

- Muscular endurance = maximum repetition pushups.

- Explosive strength = plyometric pushups, or clapping your hands between pushups.

As you build muscular strength, explosive strength also tends to increase. But to build explosive strength specifically, you need to work on it specifically. To build impressive strength; that is, strength that makes a noticeable difference, you must train against a high level of resistance. This can come in the form of weight machines, free weights, or your own bodyweight resistance.

If using bodyweight exercises, such as pushups, pull-ups, squats, and situps, or exercises that do not rely on an outside weight, you can increase the resistance by training on *uneven* surfaces. For example, place one hand higher than the other, or your feet higher than your hands for pushups. You can also increase the resistance by training on *unstable* surfaces, for example, on a stability ball for sit-ups. Training on unstable surfaces forces you to tense your muscles harder in order to keep your balance. Tightening or tensing your muscles makes it easier to control your body; in short, it makes your body function as a single unit rather than as many separate parts.

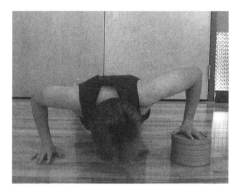

Doing pushups with one hand elevated is a great way to increase the difficulty of this bodyweight exercise. Start by placing your hand on a low obstacle, such as a weight stack. As you get stronger, increase the height of the obstacle.

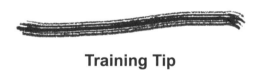

Training Tip

Many exercises train more than one muscle group at a time. For example, the pushup, if performed correctly, trains not only your upper body and arms, but also your abs and back. The squat trains not only your quadriceps, but also your hamstrings, glutes, and calves. Whenever possible, train several muscle groups at a time by using bodyweight exercises or dumbbells, rather than rigid weight machines.

Your training program

Although you need a good general strength base, your ultimate goal is not to develop general strength, but to develop specific strength that helps you outperform your opponent, whether in traditional karate, grappling, or mixed martial arts; whether in sparring, techniques, forms competition, or real self-defense. Your training program must therefore be designed for developing strength that is specific to the martial arts. Your program should have enduring qualities; you should be able to use it consistently so that it becomes habit rather than a three-week stint prior to a belt promotion or competition. A good program makes you physically able and mentally prepared to use your martial art whenever you need it. An art-specific training program on top of a good general strength base gives you the confidence to do so.

Your strength-training program should include exercises that develop your power, speed, coordination, agility, flexibility, and endurance (both muscular and cardiovascular). Which quality you develop the most depends on the specific requirements of your art. For example, if you are a Thai-boxer, great flexibility in the legs might be less crucial than if you are a Tae-Kwon-Do fighter. The type of quickness you need for grappling differs from the type of quickness you need to intercept and counter your opponent's punch. Development in one area often leads to development in another, but focusing primarily on your true needs makes you stand out as a superior fighter in your particular field.

Training often is more important than training long. If you can spend just half an hour on strength training 3 to 5 days a week, you are better off than if you go to the gym once a week and train for 4 hours straight. Frequent training conditions your body to rise to the occasion, to be ready to take on the load that lies ahead. Frequent training is a good motivator. You establish disciplined habits, and you don't have to get over the mental hurdle of going to the gym. Short duration staves off burnout.

Although you are training for strength, remember your specific reason for training: to become a better martial artist. You must continue practicing your martial art. If weight lifting seems to dominate your life, you are not training for the martial arts anymore.

Summing it up

• Our capacity for developing strength is somewhat limited by our genetic inheritance. In other words, some people have a pre-existing advantage over others that we can't do much about. But having "good genes" is only one factor that influences your ability to develop strength. A more important quality may be desire, the recognition that strength is important and will make you a better martial artist. You have now taken the first step toward starting a productive strength-training program.

• Your martial arts skill, background, and experiences are not substitutes for strength; they are complementary qualities. Martial arts practiced at a high level require strength and endurance throughout the body, not just in isolated parts.

• Your strength program should be a means to an end, and not an end in itself. Train for performance in your art, not for bigger muscles. Focus on what needs to be done and how you are doing it, and not on the maximum number of repetitions you can do in a given exercise.

• Make time for a general conditioning and fitness program to build your strength base and decrease the risk of injuries. Once such a program becomes part of you, you will start to hunger for more, for the opportunity to train even if just for 20 minutes a day. General muscular strength and endurance, flexibility, and cardiovascular fitness must be maintained at a level that you can live with.

• When you have achieved a general fitness base, analyze the particular type of strength you need in order to beat your opponent. At this stage, sport specific training plays a key role.

• If maintained over time, strength has the capacity to grow continuously; it is a gradual development influenced by the decisions you make. But training for useful strength involves more than making a gradual progression from one weight to the next. How strong you are depends on the amount of effort you expend. This includes time, intensity, and precision training relating to your particular style of martial art. What most people consider general strength, such as attending martial arts class 3 times a week, is not enough if you want to compete on a higher level. To prepare to win, you must go beyond general strength and set specific strength goals.

• Look at strength primarily as muscular strength and not as cardiovascular endurance. In other words, it is not enough to go out and run 5 miles a day. The martial arts require more than a good heart. They require explosiveness and short bursts of muscular strength; they require that you can sustain a muscular effort for a longer period of time.

• The martial arts history books are filled with accounts of tiny, fragile, and sickly men who developed the capacity to perform such astonishing feats as fending off 10 simultaneous attackers. But you can't take a historic scene, remove it from the specific times and circumstances under which it occurred, and hope to duplicate it in our modern times several centuries later. There is no easy way. If you are overweight, under-conditioned, or lazy, face this simple fact: To gain a winning edge, you must condition yourself above the basic requirements of your art, regardless of what kinds of hurdles stand in your way.

Muscle Anatomy

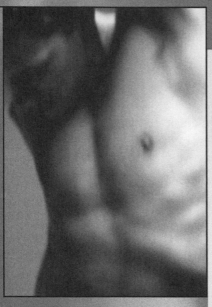

In this section:

- Types of muscle tissue

- Major muscle groups

- Types of muscle contractions

- Opposing muscle pairs

- Slow twitch, fast twitch

- Competitive advantage

- Genetic advantage

- Born or made?

Muscle Anatomy

Our main areas of study are muscular strength, muscular endurance, explosive strength, and cardiovascular endurance. Stronger muscles mean greater ability to utilize your strength, and less dead weight, such as fat, that must be lugged around. Stronger muscles mean more control over the movement of your body, and therefore better ability to manipulate your body efficiently in the martial arts. The size of bones and muscles differ between individuals, but their functions are identical.

Remember you can maintain most of your muscular strength throughout your entire life, as long as you stay active. Muscles don't atrophy as a result of age; they atrophy as a result of inactivity.

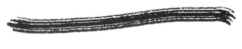

Size and Strength

Strength is measured through body composition, or muscle to fat ratio. Although physical size gives you more momentum and might therefore make you more difficult to defeat in a sparring match, it does not automatically give you more muscular strength. However, in general, a bigger person also has bigger cross-sectional areas of his muscles, and bigger cross-sectional areas generally mean greater strength.

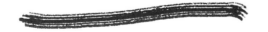

Types of muscle tissue

The human body has roughly 640 named muscles in addition to many smaller unnamed ones. These muscles are made up of several billion muscle fibers. Strength training increases the size of the muscle fibers. When the fibers grow, your muscles become stronger and can handle greater loads. This is called hypertrophy. Although the fibers grow larger with training, the number of fibers in the muscles remains the same.

Your muscles are primarily responsible for moving your body and limbs. Some muscles we have control over, and others we don't. For example, the heart muscle pumps all the time, whether we want it to or not. There are three types of muscle tissue:

- **Skeletal muscle tissue** is arranged in definite striated patterns, and is under voluntarily control. Most skeletal muscles are comprised of two types of fibers: fast-twitch and slow-twitch. In most people, one type of fiber dominates.

- **Visceral or smooth muscle tissue** is comprised of sheets or layers, and is under involuntary control. This muscle tissue is found in the walls of hollow organs, such as the stomach and digestive tract.

- **Cardiac or heart muscle tissue** is a unique tissue found only in the walls of the heart, and is under involuntary control.

The type of muscle tissue we are concerned with is skeletal tissue, which we have control over and can move and strengthen with appropriate training.

Front View of Major Muscle Groups

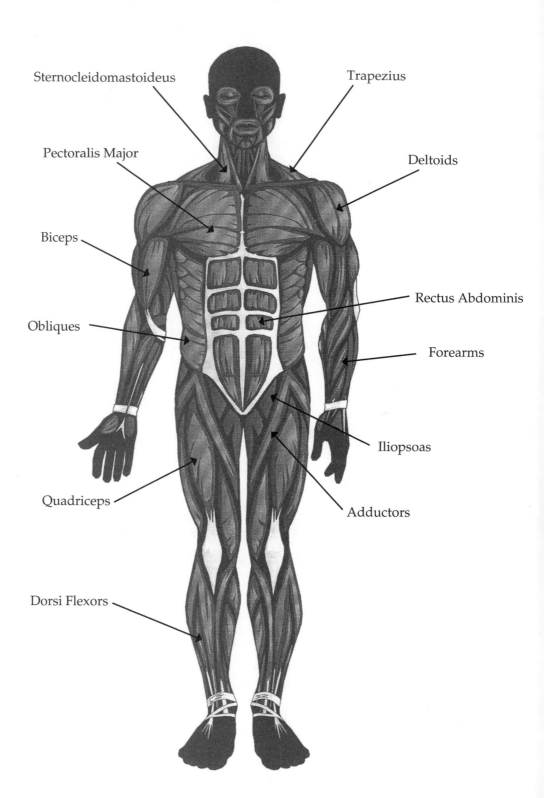

Sternocleidomastoideus

Trapezius

Pectoralis Major

Deltoids

Biceps

Rectus Abdominis

Obliques

Forearms

Quadriceps

Iliopsoas

Adductors

Dorsi Flexors

Rear View of Major Muscle Groups

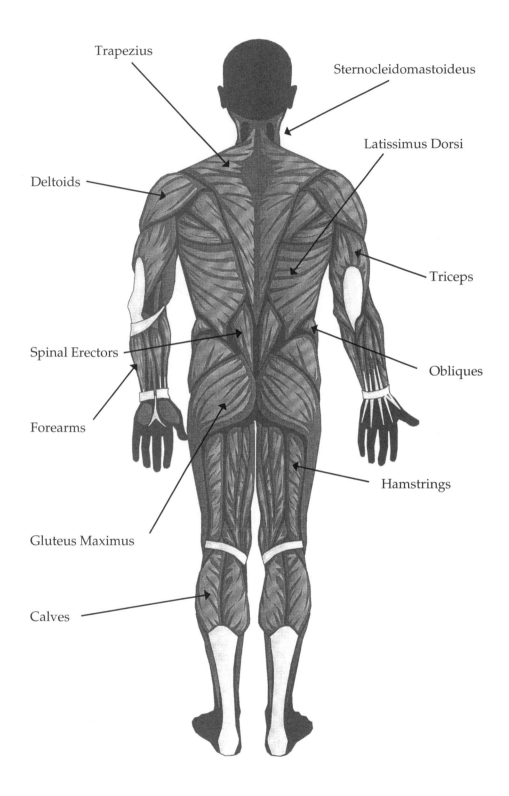

Trapezius

Sternocleidomastoideus

Deltoids

Latissimus Dorsi

Triceps

Spinal Erectors

Obliques

Forearms

Hamstrings

Gluteus Maximus

Calves

Major muscle groups

The body can be broken down into the legs, hips, abdomen and lower back, upper torso, and arms. Let's look at the major muscle groups of each section and discuss their main functions.

Legs

- **Dorsi Flexors.** This muscle group is comprised of four muscles and is located on the front of the lower leg. Its main function is to flex the foot toward the knee; for example, when throwing a sidekick impacting with the heel of the foot.

- **Calves.** This muscle group is comprised of two major muscles and is located on the back of the lower leg. Its main function is to extend the foot; for example, when throwing a roundhouse kick impacting with the instep.

- **Quadriceps.** This muscle group is comprised of four muscles and is located on the front of the thigh. Its main function is to extend or straighten the lower leg at the knee; for example, when throwing a front kick from a chambered leg position. This muscle group is also involved when walking, running, and jumping.

- **Hamstrings.** This muscle group is comprised of three muscles and is located on the back of the upper leg. Its main function is to flex the lower leg at the knee or raise the heel toward the butt; for example, when throwing a spur kick to an opponent behind you. This muscle group is also involved when walking, running, and jumping.

Hips

- **Adductors.** This muscle group is comprised of five muscles and is located along the inner thigh. Its main function is to bring the legs together; for example, when on your back in a grappling match with your opponent in your guard (between your legs).

- **Abductors.** This muscle group is located along the outer thigh. Its main function is to spread the legs; for example, when shuffling to the side.

- **Iliopsoas.** This muscle group is comprised of two primary muscles and is located on the front hip. Its main function is to flex the hip or bring the knee toward the chest; for example, when raising your leg in the chambered position in preparation for throwing a kick. This muscle group is also involved when walking, running, and climbing stairs.

- **Gluteus Maximus.** This muscle group is one of the three muscle groups that make up the buttocks, and is the largest and naturally strongest muscle group in the body. Its main function is to extend the hip or drive the leg to the rear; for example, when throwing a back or sidekick.

Abdomen and Lower Back

- **Rectus Abdominis.** This is one long muscle that extends from the lower rib cage to the pelvis. When this muscle is well developed, it looks like six or eight separate muscles, or what we normally refer to as a "six-pack" or "washboard abs." Its main function is to bring the torso toward the lower body; for example, when doing a crunch or a head butt, as discussed in Chapter 3.

• **Obliques.** This muscle group is comprised of the external and internal obliques and is located on both sides of the waist. Its main function is to bend and rotate the torso to the side, for example, when pivoting to throw or avoid a strike, or when throwing your opponent diagonally over your hip.

• **Spinal Erectors.** This is the main muscle group of the lower back. Its main function is to straighten the upper torso; for example, after you have thrown your opponent over your hip and you need to straighten your back from the bent-over position.

Upper Torso

• **Pectoralis Major.** This is the major chest muscle. Its main function is to bring the arm across the body; for example, when throwing a hook, doing an inward block, or when pushing your opponent back with your hand brought diagonally toward your centerline.

• **Latissimus Dorsi.** This is the major muscle of the upper back. Its main function is to pull the upper arm back and down, for example, when elbowing an opponent behind you and to the side, or when grabbing an opponent's hair and pulling him to the side and down.

• **Trapezius.** This is a long muscle consisting of three fiber areas that run down the upper section of the back, from the base of the skull to the middle of the lower back. Since the muscle fibers run in different directions, this muscle has several functions: to lift (for example, in a shoulder shrug), to pull down, and to pull toward the centerline of the back. A strong trapezius muscle is needed to lift your own bodyweight; for example, when climbing a rope or high fence. A strong trapezius muscle also helps you avoid neck tension headaches after performing upper body training.

• **Deltoids.** This muscle group is comprised of three muscles, and is the most important of the muscles of the shoulder. Its main function is to raise the upper arm forward, to the side, and to the rear; for example, when elbowing an opponent in front or behind you.

• **Sternocleidomastoideus** (bet you can't pronounce that!) This muscle group is comprised of two muscles on each side of the neck. Its main function is to tilt the head forward, back, and to the side, and to turn the head side-to-side. The muscles on both sides of the neck can contract together or independently. When contracting together, the head tilts toward the chest. When contracting independently, the head turns or tilts toward the shoulder. A strong neck is important in striking arts that require you to take blows to the head, or in grappling arts that use head locks or other techniques that place stress on the head or neck.

Arms

• **Biceps.** This muscle group is comprised of two muscles located on the front of the upper arm. Its main function is to bend the arm at the elbow; for example, when grabbing your opponent's lapels and pulling him toward you into a knee strike.

• **Triceps.** This muscle group is comprised of three muscles located on the back of the upper arm. Its main function is to straighten the arm at the elbow; for example, when throwing a back fist, blocking your opponent's kick with a down and outward block, or pushing your opponent back.

• **Forearms.** This muscle group is comprised of two major muscle groups containing several smaller muscles on the front and back of the forearm. Its main function is to turn the palm downward or upward; for example, when rotating the fist to the horizontal position when striking, or when applying certain joint control holds. The forearms are important in techniques that involve gripping and twisting.

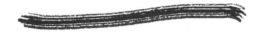

Bi, Tri, Quad, What?

The different muscle groups have derived their names from Latin. The prefix tells you something about the muscle group. For example, *bi*ceps tells you the muscle group is comprised of two muscles, *tri*ceps tells you the muscle group is comprised of three muscles, and *quad*riceps tells you the muscle group is comprised of four muscles. Compare the bi, tri, and quad prefixes to other common words indicating two, three, and four: for example, bicycle, tripod, and quarter.

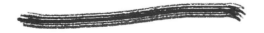

Types of muscle contractions

Muscles are comprised of flexors and extensors. The flexors bring one body part closer to another; the extensors extend one body part away from another. Muscles have only one function: to contract and pull. They cannot push. Thus, when the flexors contract, the joint bends; when the extensors contract, the joint extends. There are three types of muscle contractions:

• **Concentric Contraction.** This type of contraction happens when the muscle shortens; for example, when you do a bicep curl your biceps experience a concentric contraction. This is also called the positive phase and strengthens the muscle throughout its range of motion. Most strength training falls into this category.

• **Eccentric Contraction.** This type of contraction happens when the muscle lengthens; for example, when you lower the weight in a controlled manner. This is also called the negative phase. The same muscles are worked in concentric and eccentric contractions. Eccentric strength is always greater than concentric strength, so you can use a heavier weight during the eccentric or negative phase than during the concentric or positive phase. If you achieve muscular failure during concentric contraction, you can usually do a couple of additional reps of eccentric contraction only.

• **Isometric Contraction.** *Iso* is derived from the Greek *isos*, meaning equal. This type of contraction happens when there is no change in the length of the muscle; for example, when you hold the weight steady without raising or lowering it. Isometric contraction strengthens the muscle only at the specific angle you use in the exercise. This type of strength might be valuable in the martial arts, for example, in grappling when holding your opponent down. However, I generally don't recommend isometric training for sports, because it fails to expose your muscles to their entire range of motion. For example, when grabbing and pulling your opponent toward you, you might need strength at a distance with your arms almost straight, at mid-point with your arms bent at the elbow, and at close range. The same is true when pushing your opponent away from you. You can derive the most benefit from your training by using a combination of concentric, eccentric, and isometric lifting techniques.

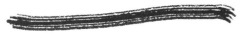

Training Tip

Negatives (eccentric contractions), or lowering the weight with control, involve the lengthening of the muscle and allow the muscle to be stretched. Take advantage of the negative phase. Do not simply drop the weight with the aid of gravity. To benefit from the negative repetition, do it slowly. About 5-8 seconds is recommended per rep.

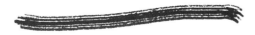

Some muscle groups have an identical antagonistic muscle; for example, the deltoids on the front and back of the shoulder, the obliques on the sides of the body, and the sternocleidomastoideus on the sides of the neck.

Opposing muscle pairs

Since your body needs to move in many different directions, the muscles usually exist in opposing pairs. When a muscle contracts and pulls, the opposite muscle relaxes. For example, the biceps to the front and the triceps to the rear of the upper arm are opposing muscle pairs. When the biceps contract, the triceps relax and your arm bends; when the triceps contract, the biceps relax and your arm straightens. On the legs, the quadriceps to the front and the hamstrings to the rear are opposing muscle pairs. The opposing muscle is referred to as the antagonistic muscle.

When strengthening our muscles, we often focus on only one muscle and fail to strengthen the antagonistic muscle. For example, we work on the pectorals (chest muscles) but not on the back. When you train one muscle group, the biceps, for example, you must also train the opposing muscle group, the triceps, in such a way that you allow them to contract and build more strength. In order to achieve a balanced set of muscles, you need to do a pulling exercise every time you do a pushing exercise, and vice versa. For example, if you do a set of pushups, it is wise to follow that with a set of seated rows.

Opposing Muscle Pairs

Dorsi Flexors – Calves
Quadriceps – Hamstrings
Adductors – Abductors
Iliopsoas – Gluteus Maximus
Rectus Abdominis – Spinal Erectors
Pectoralis Major – Trapezius
Deltoids – Latissimus Dorsi
Biceps – Triceps

Slow-twitch, fast-twitch

How well your muscles respond to strength training is influenced by a number of factors, including your particular genetics or muscle composition. The different types of muscle fibers, including their length and diameter, influence how strong you can become, how fast you can sprint, and for how long you can keep going. The muscles are comprised of slow and fast-twitch fibers, with different capacity for endurance and speed of contraction.

• **Slow-twitch** fibers are smaller in size and work primarily aerobically (with oxygen). Slow-twitch fibers are relatively fatigue resistant and have greater endurance than fast-twitch fibers. But this also means that they have less power output.

• **Fast-twitch** fibers are larger in size and work primarily anaerobically (without oxygen), and have less aerobic endurance. Fast-twitch fibers fatigue quicker than slow-twitch fibers, but have a greater power output. They are capable of more powerful contractions and therefore more explosiveness. Training with heavy loads allows you to recruit the fast-twitch fibers.

If you were born with predominantly slow-twitch muscle fibers, you are genetically predisposed for activities requiring muscular endurance. Do the martial arts require endurance? How about a 30-minute grappling match? If you were born with predominantly fast-twitch muscle fibers, you can grow big muscles easier and are genetically predisposed for activities requiring explosive strength.

It is likely that a person born with predominantly fast-twitch fibers can jump higher than a person born with predominantly slow-twitch fibers, because fast-twitch fibers contract faster than slow-twitch fibers. Whether or not this is advantageous is up for debate. You must also ask, at what expense? For example, if you have more fast-twitch fibers, it also means that you have fewer slow-twitch fibers. In addition, having the genetic capacity to throw an explosive jump kick might or might not be advantageous. It depends on the situation and on what you wish to achieve. In general, it is not necessary to throw a jump kick in order to succeed in combat; that is, unless the jump kick is a requirement of the specific art you are practicing.

Every person has a combination of slow and fast-twitch fibers, but the distribution is not the same for everybody. Also, you do not necessarily have the same distribution in all muscle groups. Thus, it is possible to have predominantly fast-twitch fibers in your legs, and predominantly slow-twitch fibers in your arms. "Because the distribution of fiber types varies from muscle to muscle, an endurance test would have to be performed for each muscle group." (A Practical Approach to Strength Training, Matt Brzycki)

You cannot increase the number of muscle fibers you were born with, nor can you change one fiber type into another fiber type, so you are somewhat limited by your genetic make-up. But you can work each fiber type to become stronger. For example, if you are born with predominantly slow-twitch fibers, you can still grow your fast-twitch fibers and improve your ability to accelerate or use explosive moves. But if you are born with predominantly fast-twitch fibers, you will have a greater capacity to grow your muscles and become stronger.

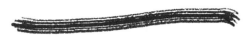

Training Tip

Explosive lifting does not translate into explosive skills in your art. Strong muscles and a large number of fast-twitch fibers translate into explosive skills. When training to increase explosiveness, use heavy loads rather than quick movement. 3-5 sets of 4-8 repetitions are recommended. If you can do more than 8 repetitions, increase the load. Make sure you are adequately rested between sets. You might want to rest as long as 3 minutes.

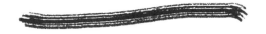

How do you know which types of muscle fibers dominate in your body? Your gut feeling probably gives you a good idea. Just look at which types of sports and activities you excel at. You can build up either type of muscle fiber, but it is easier to build the fibers that you are genetically predisposed for.

The competitive advantage

Few people would dispute that muscular strength comes from well-developed muscles. The ability to develop our muscles is partly genetic, which suggests that every person does not have the same potential to develop his or her muscles to the same degree. However, every martial artist has the potential to develop his or her muscles to some degree. If you examine elite athletes engaged in martial arts, you will see a wide variety ranging from children to the elderly, including men and women of all sizes and physical shapes. For example, Bruce Lee was relatively small in size but was probably the most famous martial artist of our time. Ken Shamrock, on the other hand, is large in size and has raked in an impressive string of wins in his mixed martial arts competitions.

Women are generally smaller than men, so it is reasonable to expect fewer variations in size and shape. Although it is true that your muscular strength is dependent on the size of your muscles, your strength is not necessarily proportional to your muscular development. Strength is not exclusively due to size. Mechanical advantages, such as limb length and tendon insertions, as well as amount of fast-twitch fibers and neural efficiency, affect strength. This is why females, for example, can have great strength without having greatly developed muscles. When considering muscle development, think in terms of muscular strength, and not in terms if muscular size.

"In general, bodybuilders are more muscular than powerlifters, but powerlifters are stronger. Studies have shown an intense set of 5 reps involves more fibers than an intense set of 1 rep. Research has shown that using loads in the 90% range causes failure to occur before a growth stimulus has been sent to the cells. Research has shown heavy lifting enhances neural efficiency, which enhances strength, but does not necessarily result in muscular growth." (www.bodybuilding.com)

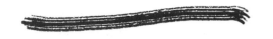

Training Tip

The intensity with which you train is the primary factor determining the growth of muscular strength. Whether you use machines, free weights, or bodyweight exercises is of less importance, as long as you use high intensity and high loads with a progressive schedule that fatigues the muscles. To develop muscular strength, use high loads and few repetitions, between 4 and 8 reps per set. If you can do more, increase the load.

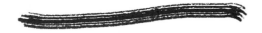

The genetic advantage

Your genetic inheritance directly affects how successful you are at your sport and how you respond to strength training, and plays a key role in your ability to develop muscle size and strength. This includes factors such as your weight, height, muscle composition, and mental state. Some of these factors you cannot change, for example, your height. Others you can change, at least to a degree, for example, your weight. You must therefore learn to make the most of those qualities that you cannot change, and train to strengthen the others. For example, if you are naturally flexible, more training can help you reach kicking heights on the elite level. Let's look at the key genetic factors:

Body Type

Body type refers to your body composition. This includes the length of your bones, the length and width of your upper body, and your lean mass to fat ratio. Lean mass includes bone, muscle, and connective tissue. There are thee kinds of body types:

• **Endomorph.** This body type is characterized by a high percentage of body fat, little muscle definition, and rounded features. People with this body type generally fall into the category of being slower and less agile than others. However, the fact that the muscles aren't well defined does not necessarily mean that this body type lacks significant muscle; rather, the muscles are hidden by layers of fat. This body type therefore has the potential to exercise considerable strength. A Sumo wrestler is an example of an endomorph.

• **Ectomorph.** This body type is characterized by a low percentage of body fat, long limbs, and a slender build. Ectomorphs lack thick muscle bellies but can still have considerable muscle definition, due to the low amount of body fat. However, in general, this body type does not lend itself to great muscular development and strength. A marathon runner is an example of an ectomorph.

• **Mesomorph.** This body type is characterized by mostly lean body tissue, broad shoulders, a slim waistline, and a heavily muscled physique. This body type has a great potential for developing muscular size and strength. An example of a true mesomorph is a competitive bodybuilder.

Those at the far end of the spectrum can respectively be thought of as fat, lean, and muscular. Although most people have a tendency toward one body type, few fall at the extreme end. Most of us fall somewhere in-between these categories and have qualities that overlap.

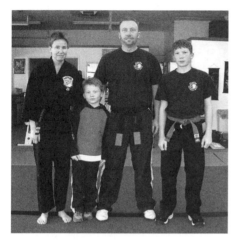

Men and women of all ages and body types practice the martial arts and need strong muscles to succeed.

Bone Length

The length of your bones, and therefore the length of your limbs, gives you strength qualities through biomechanical leverage. A person with long arms and legs must present a greater effort than a person with short arms and legs. For example, in pushing and pulling moves, short arms give you a strength advantage over long arms, because you don't have to move the weight as far. A person with short arms has therefore an easier time with pushups or bench presses. The same applies to short vs. long legs. A person with short legs will seem stronger than a person with long legs in squatting or leg press exercises; again, because the weight is moved over a shorter

distance. In pushing and pulling moves, the biomechanical advantage goes to the person with short levers. However, if your martial art does not rely mainly on pushing or pulling moves, longer arms and legs might give you a different advantage, such as the ability to cover distance quicker.

Muscle-to-Tendon Ratio

The potential for muscular growth is related to the muscle belly to tendon ratio. Tendons connect muscle to bone. The muscle belly is located between the two attachment points of the tendon. If you have a long muscle belly and a short tendon, you have a greater capacity for developing muscular size, than if you have a short muscle belly and a long tendon. You can compare the lengths of your muscle bellies with those of your martial arts friends. The muscle bellies on the biceps, triceps, and calves are the easiest to see.

Tendon Insertion Points

Some people appear to have considerable strength without significant muscular development. A reason for this may be a biomechanical advantage derived from the insertion points of the tendons, or the attachment point of the tendon on the bone. The farther the tendon inserts from the axis of rotation, the greater the strength advantage. For example, if you are doing a bicep curl, you will have a biomechanical advantage if the bicep tendon attaches an inch down the forearm, rather than closer to the crook of the elbow.

Muscle Cross-Sectional Area

Muscle cross-sectional area can be related to the mass of the muscle. A big muscle has a large cross-sectional area. A large cross-sectional area contains a greater number of protein filaments and has a greater capacity to generate force, so a large cross-sectional area is always accompanied with an improvement in relative strength. A long muscle belly is generally an indication that there is a large cross-sectional area.

Neurological Efficiency

Neurological efficiency is the measure of how quickly your central nervous system can recruit muscle fibers. Some people can recruit a higher percentage of their muscle fibers than others, which gives them a greater potential for strength. The quicker the fibers are activated, and the greater the percentage of fibers activated, the greater the speed and strength of the muscle. Neurological efficiency is inversely proportional to anaerobic muscle endurance (which is not the same as cardiovascular endurance). In simple terms, this means that some people have a greater capacity for developing muscular strength, and others have a greater capacity for developing muscular endurance.

Testosterone

Finally, testosterone levels affect your muscles' potential for hypertrophy and are your body's natural muscle building hormones. When these growth hormones are stimulated through exercise, muscular growth occurs. Testosterone level is an inherited trait, and is one reason men have greater capacity than women for developing muscular size.

Born or made?

Because of the genetic factor, a common subject of debate is whether great athletes are born or made. My opinion is that great athletes, in any field, are mainly born. This doesn't mean that all you have to do is look at a stranger and tell whether he or she is a great athlete. For example, a big or stocky person is not automatically a good wrestler, nor is a skinny person with long arms automatically a quick puncher. There are many others factors that contribute to success in your sport; for example, time and intensity of training, strategy and skill development, and your mental state. Genetics alone do not guarantee that you will improve your strength or your martial arts skill.

Without the right training, you cannot bring out superior qualities. Other than genetics, the most determining factor is intensity of training. Lack of intensity, or failing to work your muscles to fatigue, results in little strength gain. Motivation is also a key factor. Motivation is the driving force that allows you to build on the physical qualities you are born with. If a person with all the genetic advantages is not disciplined in his or her training, the competitive advantage goes to the less strong but more disciplined athlete. To benefit the most from motivation, it must originate with you, and not with your parents, your spouse, or your friends. There are no substitutes for hard work, tenacity, and commitment. To become an elite athlete, you must have a combination of the right genetic inheritance, learned skills in your art, a strong and healthy body, and a strong mind.

take advantage of biomechanical principles, supplements weight lifting and helps you gain a greater strength benefit.

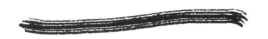

Genetic Excellence

Many athletes choose their sports based on their genetic capabilities. In short, we choose a sport in which we have a natural tendency to excel. As we experiment with playing sports as youngsters, we discover where we excel. This creates a chain reaction: When we do well, we participate more often, which leads to development of better skills in areas where we are already strong, which allows us to excel even more. This is also why so many basketball players are tall. They didn't grow tall as a result of playing basketball; rather, they realized that their height would help them excel at their game. The tallest athletes choose to play basketball, the fastest athletes choose sprinting, and the strongest athletes choose wrestling or power lifting. Mental strength and balance, as required in the martial arts, is also a genetic quality. Is it possible that some of us choose the martial arts based on our inherited genetic mental qualities?

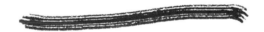

Before we move on and develop our strength training routines, let's look at how to maximize strength through the use of Natural Anatomical Strengths (Chapter 3), and Physics and Biomechanical Strengths (Chapter 4). When you perform your techniques in accordance with these laws, you achieve the greatest results with the least amount of energy expenditure. Knowledge of human anatomy, its strengths and weaknesses, and knowledge of how to

Natural Anatomical Strengths

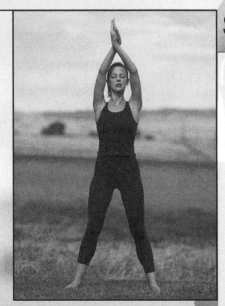

In this section:

- Injury prevention

- The skeletal system

- The fist

- Striking mechanics

- Kicking mechanics

- Blocking mechanics

- Pivot and alignment

- The head butt

- Water and sweat

Natural Anatomical Strengths

Karate and other forms of unarmed combat enable the practitioners to deliver blows of devastating power. But if the techniques are improperly applied, or if the practitioner lacks understanding of how to use the human anatomy to his or her advantage, injury is often the price. You must therefore have knowledge of the body's natural strengths and limitations. The movements of hands, feet, body, and neck are not independent of each other, but should be synchronized in such a way that they can draw from and support each other in strength and speed. Studying the anatomy and structure of the human body helps you acquire a more complete understanding of movement capabilities for offense and defense.

Natural strengths and injury prevention

Some parts of your anatomy can withstand the demands of your art better than other parts. For example, it is better to use the fleshy rather than the bony part of your forearm when blocking a strike. Understanding your natural strengths and weaknesses helps you use the stronger body parts to take the impact of blows, or at least identify which parts of your body need to be conditioned further. Strength and injury avoidance are also determined through proper joint and bone alignment. A good understanding of your anatomy can help you maximize the use of your body's muscles and joints. Try this:

- Stand sideways on one leg on a grassy slope. Stand on the uphill foot first and pay attention to where the pressure is. Then stand on the downhill foot and compare.

- When on the uphill foot, the pressure should be toward the inside of your foot; when on the downhill foot, the pressure should be toward the outside of your foot. Most people are built so that they are naturally stronger toward the outside knife-edge of the foot than toward the inside knife-edge.

- If kicking when standing on a sloping surface, you are stronger if you kick with your uphill foot and use your downhill foot for support, than vice versa. Having an idea of your natural anatomical strengths helps you utilize them to your advantage as often as possible.

The skeletal system

The skeletal system supports the human body and is comprised of a total of 206 bones that are connected by joints. Because of the symmetry of the body, most bones exist in pairs. The primary function of the bones of the torso is to protect the internal organs. The primary function of the bones of the extremities is to support your weight and provide movement of the arms and legs. More than half of the 206 bones are found in the extremities. Since we use the arms and legs for striking, kicking, blocking, and grabbing, these are the bones we will discuss in this chapter.

The ligaments stabilize the joints and limit their range of motion. Going against the natural range of motion of a joint

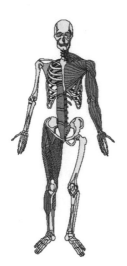

increases the risk of injury to that joint. The range of motion is determined by the joint structure, the thickness of the tissue, and the strength of the ligaments.

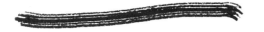

Bone Breaking Tough

Bones can withstand an incredible amount of pressure. In a 125-pound person, some parts of the femur (thigh bone) routinely withstand pressures of 1200 pounds per square inch just through the daily activity of walking. However, the bones can withstand direct pressure better than force caused by rotation. Since many martial arts techniques require body rotation in order to maximize power and follow-through, you must synchronize body movements to minimize the risk of injury during the execution of the technique.

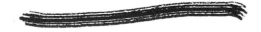

The fist

The most common striking weapon is the fist because it is naturally fast and precise. But the joints of the hand are sensitive to injury, and include the wrist and knuckles on the fingers and hand. The more solid the fist is, the less likely you are to injure it. Injury prevention also applies to how straight you impact the target. When striking, clench your fist tightly to eliminate any gap between your hand and fingers that can cause the fist to "collapse" on impact. Keep your wrist straight in both the horizontal and vertical plane to ensure that the bones of the forearm are properly aligned to absorb the force. Impacting the target with the knuckles of the first two fingers ensures proper straightness of the wrist.

There has been some debate as to whether the fist should be rotated to the horizontal position on impact, or if it is better to strike with the fist in the vertical position. When holding the fist in the vertical position (thumb up), the ulna and radius bones of the forearm are parallel. When turning the fist to the horizontal position palm down, the two bones of the forearm cross, possibly lessening their ability to absorb the force. Striking with a vertical fist may therefore be stronger.

Striking mechanics and injury prevention

The ulna and radius bones should be parallel for maximum strength.

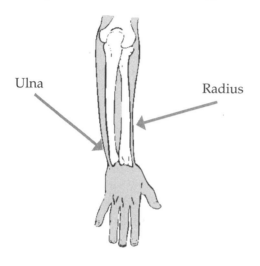

Ulna

Radius

When the bones, tendons, ligaments, and muscles are aligned, the strike is capable of generating more power with a reduction in the likelihood of injury to the practitioner. However, the hand position that feels most natural is generally also the strongest. Since everybody has slightly different preferences regarding striking in the martial arts, in order to find what works for you, some experimentation must take place beyond a theoretical understanding.

In order to strike a target without risking injury, the force of the striking weapon must transfer into the target. Power is generated through a strong and balanced stance. Relaxing and tensing at the proper time is important. If you clench your fists too tightly and you miss, you waste energy and may lose your balance. The synchronization of your legs, hips, shoulders, and back is essential to powerful and injury free striking.

Most martial artists are familiar with the concepts of leg strength and hip rotation, but seldom do we discuss the importance our back serves in the execution and absorption of blows. The back is the connection between your stance, or foundation, and your strikes. If your back is swayed or not properly aligned, your balance and strength are affected and you lack the momentum to strike with penetrating force. This also applies to defense: Your back should be straight and your hips slightly tucked in order to absorb the force of a strong push or blow.

When you have achieved proper stance and body alignment, choose specific targets with care to maximize the effectiveness of the strike and minimize the risk of injury to the striking weapon. Time the strike to impact the target slightly before your arm is fully extended. If the strike impacts at the precise moment of the full extension of your arm, your own body absorbs the force instead of the target you are striking.

The "non-striking" side of your body should assist the striking side for maximum power, speed, and target penetration. Many of us focus only on the hand that is doing the striking. Although we use proper rotation in the feet and hips, we tend to neglect the use of the upper body, especially the non-striking hand. You can increase the power of your strikes by pivoting your body and pulling back your non-striking hand simultaneous with the forward motion of your striking hand. The movements between your hands should be coordinated for maximum efficiency. Failing to do this creates a contradiction in the direction of energy; kind of like stepping on the gas pedal and the brake simultaneously when driving your car.

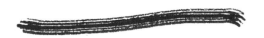

Punching Air

Because of the lack of a target, a greater risk of injury exists when punching air in training. When you snap your arm straight in the air, your own body (shoulder and elbow) provides the stopping motion and therefore absorbs the full force of the blow. When striking the air during warm-up or practice, exercise caution and slow the strike gradually to avoid hyperextension of the elbow or shoulder.

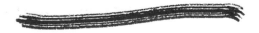

Let's look at natural anatomical strengths and injury prevention for a number of popular karate strikes.

Shuto (knife hand strike or chop)

The weaknesses of the hand are in the little finger and wrist. The force must therefore be absorbed by the fleshy part of the hand between the little finger and wrist, and not with the fingers or wrist themselves. Impacting too close to the wrist may result in injury to the wrist or ulna bone; impacting too close to the fingers may result in injury to the knuckle or ligaments of the little finger. Since the shuto often impacts at an angle from the side, keeping your elbow slightly bent allows you to use the weight of your body to increase the power of the blow without risking injury to your elbow. For example, if you throw an outward shuto (away from your centerline) with full extension of the arm, which results in a locked elbow on impact, the elbow provides at least some of the stopping motion and absorbs some of the force. The risk of injury therefore increases. If you throw an outward shuto with a slightly bent arm and body rotation for follow-through, the force on the elbow is decreased.

Ridge Hand Strike (reverse shuto or chop)

This strike employs similar striking mechanics to the shuto, but impacts with the fleshy part of the hand between the wrist and first knuckle of the index finger. The thumb must be tucked into the palm of the hand to avoid impacting with the knuckles of the thumb.

Heel Palm Strike

This is a strong blow that utilizes the fleshy part of the hand on the little finger side of the palm itself. When striking with the heel palm, be careful not to impact with the wrist. A slight bend in the elbow on impact allows the arm to absorb the power of the strike.

Fingers

Although smaller jointed and weaker than the hand, the fingers can still be used as effective striking weapons. When using the fingers for striking and poking, make sure the fingers are not bent backwards against their natural range of motion. Finger strikes should be used primarily against soft tissue areas that can be penetrated, such as the eyes or throat. If using a roundhouse blow, bend the fingers slightly at the knuckles in the hand to decrease the risk of injury to the hand. You can also use a single finger when striking smaller targets such as the eyes, with the other fingers folded into the palm of your hand. Again, to decrease the risk of injury to your hand, bend the striking finger slightly inward.

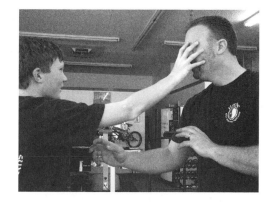

Your fingers are small-jointed and relatively weak. To avoid injury, bend your fingers slightly and strike to a target that is inherently weak; for example, to your opponent's eyes.

Hammerfist Strike

Although not a sharp blow, the hammerfist is a powerful blow that is executed with a tight fist and a bent elbow, using your body weight for power. Bending the elbow places the strike closer to your body, allowing you to use bodyweight when dropping the strike into the target. The hammerfist can be dropped from above, or from a side position with a pivot in your hips and a drop in bodyweight for follow-through.

Forearm Strike

Both the inside and outside of the forearm are good striking and blocking weapons. Impact the target with the fleshy part of the forearm and not with the bone itself. When using the outside forearm strike (away from your centerline), keep your arm slightly bent on impact to avoid hyperextension of the elbow. The inside forearm strike (toward your centerline) can be used in conjunction with body momentum; for example, as a strike to your opponent's chest or upper body in preparation for a rear takedown. Do not snap your elbow into the locked position on impact.

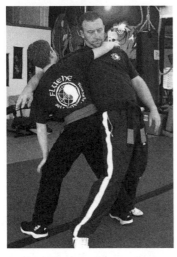

The forearm is a powerful weapon that can be used as a strike or in preparation for a takedown. Avoid striking with the bony part of the arm.

Elbow Strike

This may well be the most devastating weapon used in empty hand combat. The elbow is very small, sharp, and strong, allowing the practitioner to focus the power over a small surface area. The elbow is also closer to the shoulder than is the hand, and much of the power is generated with the weight of the heavier body behind the blow. When dropping the elbow straight down, strike with the point of the elbow itself. If dropping the elbow straight down for the purpose of breaking wood or bricks, it is

recommended that you impact the target approximately one inch above the elbow rather than with the point of the elbow to avoid injury. When using the elbow strike in a horizontal fashion (elbow sandwich), impact the target with the elbow and an inch or two down the forearm. The sweeping motion of the horizontal elbow prevents you from impacting with the point alone.

Kicking mechanics and injury prevention

Kicks are generally more awkward to throw than strikes, due to the fact that the legs are our foundation and the legs are much heavier than our arms. But with practice comes the ability to utilize the legs as weapons. The leg may be the strongest weapon you possess in empty hand combat. Another benefit of the leg is that it can be used to attack from a greater distance.

Front Kick

The most popular and easy to learn kick is perhaps the front kick, impacting the target with the ball of your foot (the fleshy portion just below your toes). Bend your toes back in order to avoid injury to your foot. Just as you must keep your wrist straight when punching, you must keep your ankle straight when kicking. A bent ankle or a "floppy" foot cannot withstand the force of impact.

Roundhouse Kick

This is another highly popular kick in most martial arts. When striking with the instep (the top portion of the foot), tuck your toes under to ensure that the instep is tight (like a springboard). Again, a foot that is floppy on impact lacks penetrating force and increases the risk of injury.

"Our feet transport most of us more than 100,000 miles in a lifetime – equal to about four trips around the world. Women generally average 10 miles a day, outdistancing men who walk an average of seven miles a day. With each step taken by a person weighing 130 pounds, the foot absorbs 500 pounds of pressure, which comes to about 5 million pounds of impact on the feet in an average day." (www.arthritis.org)

My personal feel is that most of us don't walk quite that far every day. But the point is, over a lifetime, our feet have to take a huge amount of punishment.

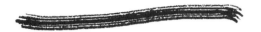

Our feet are primarily designed for bearing weight. The foot contains 26 bones, 33 joints, 107 ligaments, 19 muscles, and tendons that hold the structure together. The 52 bones in your two feet make up about one-fourth of all the bones in your body. With this in mind, the instep is not the most structurally sound impact weapon.

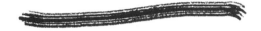

Sidekick

The sidekick impacts the target with the heel of the foot. It is a strong kick with the power derived from the small surface area of the heel, and from the big muscle of the buttocks. When impacting the target, curl your toes back and extend your heel toward the target. You can also kick a bigger target, impacting with the entire bottom portion of your foot. But this gives you less penetrating force. Since the sidekick requires considerable turn in the hips, a common mistake when throwing this kick is *under rotation*, which causes impact with the ball or toes of the foot instead of the heel. This can cause injury to your toes or ankle.

Outside Knife-Edge of Foot

This is a popular karate weapon used to attack the front, side, or back of your opponent's knees, shins, floating ribs, or throat. The outside knife-edge must be properly aligned with your leg and hip for power and injury prevention. Angle your foot in the sidekick position to avoid injury to your toes.

Sweep

The sweep is used for taking your opponent off balance or disrupting his focus. However, improper sweeping technique increases the risk of injury to your foot. When sweeping "boot-to-boot" and impacting with the inside knife-edge of your foot, it is recommended that you use the arch of your foot instead of the edge because of the greater padding of this part of the foot. This requires the sole of the foot to face slightly upward when sweeping.

Shin

Higher up the leg is the shin, which can be used as a striking weapon in the front or roundhouse kick motion. The shin is structurally stronger than the instep and is therefore a powerful weapon. But most people lack sufficient padding on the shin and are uncomfortable with even the slightest contact. When impacting with the shin, impact with the muscle that is slightly to the outside of the bone and not directly with the bone itself. If you are a kickboxer or Muay Thai fighter, a good exercise for building muscular shins is hiking uphill.

Knee

The knee is, just like the elbow, a very strong and highly effective weapon that is used primarily from close range. You can impact with the kneecap itself in a front kick motion, or with the entire thigh area in a roundhouse motion.

Blocking mechanics and injury prevention

Defense is not passive. The strength in defense lies in transforming every block into an offensive weapon. You can use your elbow, forearm, or portions of your hand for blocking, as well as your shin or foot. Avoid using the weak parts of your anatomy, which include your joints, or directly against the bone where there is little padding. An exception may be the elbow when dropped straight down on an opponent's toes, instep, ankle, or shin. Impacting with the point of the elbow is highly effective, because the small surface area of the block allows you to focus the power for sharp penetration. The target is also more prone to injury than is the elbow, so the weakest will give.

Forearm

When blocking with the forearm, use the muscular and fleshy area close to the elbow rather than the area close to the wrist. Impact close to your opponent's wrist, where he is anatomically weak.

Hand

Whenever the motion of the block goes against the natural bend of the arm, you must keep a slight bend in the elbow on impact to avoid hyperextension or full absorption of power (stopping motion), should the target suddenly be removed. If using the palm of the hand to block, keep a slight bend in the elbow at impact to allow your joints to absorb the shock without injury.

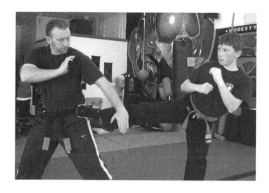

When blocking your opponent's kick in an outward motion, a slight bend in your elbow helps prevent injury.

Foot

When using your foot to block your opponent's kick, use the same motion as you would when kicking. In other words, do not block with the side of your foot where it is anatomically weak, or with your ankle. For example, when you see your opponent raise his foot to throw a front kick, intercept his kick with yours and block it by front kicking his shin before his kick is extended. Obviously, this requires timing. Using the hands for blocking is therefore easier, because the hands are quicker and more precise than the legs. But interfering with your opponent's kicks, especially from close range, gives you a physical and mental strategic advantage.

Knee

The knee is a strong defensive weapon that can be used to block a front or sidekick. Bring your knee up high, simultaneously pushing your hips forward to stifle the attack.

Pivot and leg/body alignment

Now that we have discussed the specific striking, kicking, and blocking weapons, let's discuss proper alignment of the leg with the rest of the body during the dynamic execution of a kick. Pivoting on your supporting leg allows your hips to rotate for the extension of power through the target. The question is: How much should you pivot? Is more necessarily better, or are there drawbacks to pivoting too much or too little?

Strength and injury prevention depend on correct pivots. If you don't pivot enough, you will place stress on the ankle and knee joint of your supporting leg. Remember, the joints are the weaker parts of your anatomy especially when a move involves twisting. If you pivot too much, a similar problem occurs because the ankle, knee, and hip joint are not properly aligned. Pivoting too much stresses the knee, especially if you carry a lot of bodyweight and momentum on that leg. As a guideline when pivoting, line up the toes of your supporting leg with your ankle and knee. Do not twist your foot with your toes pointed in or out.

Proper pivot gives you better balance and allows you to see the target without blocking your view with part of your own body. For example, if you pivot too much with the roundhouse kick, you are forced to view the target directly over your shoulder, which could strain your back. Without proper pivot, your kick will lack power and could cause severe damage to the joint of your supporting leg.

Case study on the head butt

According to the laws of physics, you cannot strike something without being struck back equally hard by the target you are striking.

**Newton's Third Law of Motion:
To every action there is an equal and opposite reaction.**

When two objects collide, both experience the same amount of force. So when choosing our striking weapon, we must ensure that it is structurally stronger than the target we are impacting. This is easy when using a structurally strong weapon against an inherently weak target (your stronger fist or foot against your opponent's weaker nose or knee, for example). But what if you use a specific weapon against an identical target, as is the case with the head butt? When using your head to impact your opponent's head, whose head will prevail?

Since the neck is a part of our anatomy that is easily damaged through movement, whether twisting or bouncing, we must be careful to avoid any abrupt head movements. For example, snapping the head can cause whiplash injury, even if there is no actual impact to the head. This is seen in automobile accidents where there is a quick halt in momentum. When head butting our opponent, we must therefore avoid movement in the neck. This is when your abdominal strength will assist you. First, lock your neck muscles tight so that your head and body become one unit. Use your abdominal muscles and do a standing crunch, like a quick and short bow. This places the stress on your abdomen and not on your neck muscles alone.

You must also consider the part of the head you use for impacting the target. It is obviously better to use the top portion of your skull (above and to the outside of the eyes) against a weaker part of your opponent's head (the face, nose, or between the eyes), than the other way around.

Next, consider your opponent's movement. Whereas an opponent who "walks into" your strike or kick can add power to your strike, you must be cautious with this same concept when head butting since the brain is more sensitive to serious injury than is the hand or foot. The head butt should be used primarily at short range when your hands are tied up, and not when there is a lot of momentum, as when closing distance from long range.

Water and sweat

Once you understand the strengths and weaknesses of the particular parts of your anatomy that are used for striking, kicking, and blocking, you must also know how to maintain an energy supply for these parts, mainly through controlled regulation of fluid and temperature. I will keep my discussion brief and restrict it to the two fluids that we have ability to control, namely water and sweat.

Water is the essence of life. More than 75 percent of the human body is comprised of fluids, so there is no wonder that water and sweat are important in order to keep us going at maximum efficiency. During exercise, the body is dependent on fluid to carry off excess heat in the form of sweat. The primary purpose of sweating is to allow your body to cool down. An efficient cooling system helps you last longer and recover faster between exercises.

Now, I am going to give you a test:

1. Does it benefit the martial artist to drink before, during, and after workouts?
2. Is it possible to overdose on water?

If you answered "yes" to both questions, you are right. It is important that you drink plenty of fluids before, during, and after exercise. Don't deprive yourself of drinking during exercise. Drinking does not make you a sissy athlete, but allows your body to function at maximum capacity. Drinking prevents dehydration or premature fatigue. Restricting or frowning on water consumption during workouts is a sign of the old school. Getting dehydrated during training, or training in too hot temperatures, could result in heat exhaustion and in severe cases death. Understand that fluid intake is important. Heed the warning signals.

So if drinking is good for you, then how is it possible to overdose? And how do you know if you have overdosed? In general, overdosing on water is very difficult and requires you to drink 4 to 6 quarts in a time period of one to two hours. However, overdosing on water could kill you. When your body receives too much water, the salt in the blood is diluted, causing swelling in the brain and resulting in dizziness, headache, nausea, confusion, convulsions, coma, and death. Several deaths have occurred among marathon runners and boot camp military recruits who drank a lot of water during long marches. "An Ironman competitor finished the triathlon -- swimming 2.4 miles, cycling 112 miles, and running 26.2 miles -- while drinking about 55 pounds of water in the 14 hours and three minutes it took him to cover the course. He collapsed with seizures but survived after an eight-day hospital stay." (www.usatoday.com)

The bad news is that the symptoms of overdosing are similar to the symptoms of dehydration. The good news is that overdosing on water is very difficult, and that you are far more likely not to drink enough than to drink too much. A good rule of thumb for endurance athletes is drinking about 8 to 16 ounces of water, or one medium size glass, per hour of exercise.

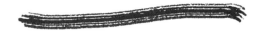

Water Intoxication

The *Annuals of Internal Medicine* reports that 18% of marathon runners drink too much water. Overdosing on water is called *hyponatremia*. When you drink too much water, vital minerals such as sodium are washed from the body. Sodium is an electrolyte that helps the body distribute water. Instead of drinking pure water during strenuous exercise, try Gatorade or other sports drinks containing salt.

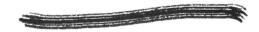

Here is the next test:

1. Is sweating a lot during training a sign of good or bad health? Why?
2. What is the purpose of sweat?

Many people are embarrassed about sweating, but it should make you proud because it is a sign of good health. Sweating a lot means that your body has an effective cooling system. In fact, you may find that as the years go by and you get in better shape, your body will adjust and start sweating more.

The purpose of sweat is to cool the body as the sweat changes state from a liquid to a gas. Energy is required to evaporate the sweat from your skin, and this energy comes from your body in the form of heat. So when the sweat evaporates, your temperature is lowered. You will feel cooler and be able to function more efficiently. This is also why you get cold the moment you step out of the lake even if the air temperature is warmer than the water you were swimming in, and even if you weren't cold when you were in the water.

Of course, sweating or allowing water to evaporate from your body when your temperature is normal or low is a bad idea and may result in hypothermia, but this is normally not the case when training for athletics.

Conclusion

Proper strength training leads to impressive changes in your body's ability to cope with the stress of the martial arts. It also leads to improved performance. Through strength training, the body adapts to the increased demands placed upon it. These adaptations include cardiovascular function, muscular endurance and muscular strength, stronger bones, and increased flexibility in tendons and ligaments. But strength training is also a process that must be accomplished gradually. The key to success in toughening the body lies in time and practice.

It is not "all in the technique." Keeping yourself in shape will help you dish it out and take it without risking undue injury.

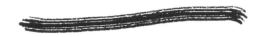

Stronger?

In today's age of low carb diets, keep in mind that these diets weren't designed for athletes. The athlete needs carbohydrates for energy, while proteins are needed mostly to repair tissue and build muscle. Without energy, you can't train hard, so the proteins won't have much to build or repair. When we talk about carbohydrates, we mean complex carbohydrates that you find in pasta, rice, vegetables, and potatoes, and not simple carbohydrates that you find in white sugar.

Since the primary purpose of this book is on how to gain strength for martial arts using a variety of muscle building exercises, and not on how to eat right, lose weight, or look good, we will not discuss proper eating habits or dietary supplements. For detailed information on this subject, please refer to *The Fighter's Body*, by Loren Christensen and Wim Demeere. Suffice it to say that carbohydrates are your body's fuel, and cutting the carbs or going on a low carb diet is not recommended for those involved in heavy physical activity.

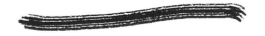

Physics and Biomechanical Strengths

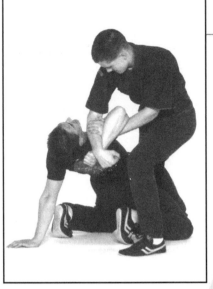

In this section:

- **Advantages in balance and motion**

- **Weighted objects and neuromuscular confusion**

- **Biomechanical efficiency**

Physics and Biomechanical Strengths

Physics and biomechanical principles have less to do with raw muscular strength, or the type of strength you develop in the weight training gym, and more to do with your apparent strength when engaged in the martial arts. A large part of biomechanics involves the study of muscular activity, and how your bones, muscles, and joints affect movement. Factors that must be considered are your physical build, such as the stockiness or slenderness of your body, your height to weight ratio, and the length of your limbs.

• **Biomechanics** is the study of the body during performance. It is the science of mechanical principles applied to biological functions, or the application of mechanics (how to gain a mechanical advantage) on living systems, such as a human being engaged in athletics. Faulty biomechanics can have a negative effect on performance and can lead to injury.

• **Physics**, or the laws of physics, sort of go hand-in-hand with biomechanics and affect how you can best utilize your muscular strength against natural forces, such as gravity, momentum, and inertia. For a more detailed study of physics and the natural laws of motion, please refer to *Fighting Science: The Laws of Physics for Martial Artists*, by Martina Sprague.

Your strength is partly a measure of your ability to apply physics and biomechanical principles to your martial art. Having a good understanding of physics and biomechanics allows you to maximize your strength, avoid wasted motion, and become a more efficient fighter.

Let's take a look at the types of movements to which these principles are applied in the martial arts.

Advantages in balance and motion

In addition to your anatomical build, your overall physical strength depends on several factors, including your mass (weight), balance, explosiveness, ability to drive off the ground (strength of your foundation), and ability to train scientifically and utilize physics and biomechanics.

A forceful fighter is often considered a strong fighter, and being muscularly strong always works to your advantage. But force and muscular strength don't necessarily coincide. In other words, a less muscularly strong fighter can still produce significant force by using physics and biomechanical principles correctly, and an already muscularly strong fighter can maximize his force by adding these principles to the equation.

By the same token, a muscularly strong fighter who fails to take advantage of these principles will appear less strong than he is. Taking advantage of the natural laws of motion allows you to conserve energy for a time during the fight or demonstration when using your maximum strength is crucial. For example, a fighter who can deadlift twice as much as his opponent in a non-threatening situation prior to a bout, may become completely worthless strength-wise when minutes into the match all his resources have been inappropriately spent. Raw physical strength is therefore no guarantee that you will persevere over an opponent of less physical strength. Using physics and correct body mechanics can make you appear stronger than your muscles or true physical capacity really allow.

When practicing the martial arts, you deal primarily with principles that affect your balance and motion. You need physics and biomechanics for:

• **Stability**, or the degree of control you have over your stability. For example, when you throw a strike or kick, a stable stance gives your strike more power than if you are off balance. When you throw your opponent over your shoulder or hip, stability helps you avoid going down with him.

• **Coordination**, or how coordinated body mechanics affect your power and, therefore, your apparent strength.

• **Transfer of strength** from one body part to another, for example, when using the strength of your legs to increase the power of a strike.

• **State of motion**, including standstill, forward, backward, upward, downward, spinning, and to the side; for example, when taking advantage of your opponent's motion in order to evade an attack and take him off balance.

• **Resistance to motion**, also called inertia, or how to minimize resistance when starting or stopping motion, when getting up from the ground, or when stopping an opponent who is tackling you.

• **Timing**, or how the force you exert over time affects your power and the damage you can inflict on your opponent

through the proper measure and use of distance.

• **Continuous or rotational motion**, for example, when increasing power by throwing combination strikes or spinning techniques.

Before we delve into the specifics of physics and biomechanics, let's talk about the difference between developing muscular strength and improving your martial arts techniques, and what type of strength training DOES NOT help improve your techniques.

Weighted objects and neuromuscular confusion

Every time you go to martial arts class, you warm up by throwing a hundred punches and kicks in the air, the same punches and kicks you have been throwing over and over for years. By doing this, you develop *neuromuscular efficiency*, or how efficiency of movement affects performance. This is why a technique begins to feel "natural" when you have done it a large number of times.

In order to develop sport specific skills, the movement you do in your strength-training program must be *identical*, not just similar, to the movement used in your martial art. For example, using weighted objects while performing sport specific moves, such as kicks, does not develop sport specific qualities; it does not make you a better kicker. You do not become a stronger and more explosive kicker by using ankle weights when practicing kicks. This is because you are changing the timing with which these kicks must be performed.

If you want to develop strong and explosive kicks, you must develop strong muscles. Remember, you develop strong muscles by using heavy weights or high intensity training. A weighted object, such as an ankle weight, is normally not heavy enough to really help you develop muscular strength. Using weighted objects could actually be adversarial to your skill, because when you take them off, your timing and accuracy are likely to have changed. If you feel as though your legs are faster after removing the weight, it is likely due to a sensory illusion rather than actual speed, because you were kicking slower against the wrong type of resistance while you were wearing the weights.

"Doing a throwing motion with a weighted wall pulley will NOT give you a better fastball pitch any more than running with heavy ankle weights will give you a faster stride. Indeed, your skill level in pitching or running would dwindle somewhat by employing these respective lifting techniques!" (Popular Training Systems: Are They Really "Systems?" Frederick C. Hatfield, Ph.D., MSS, International Sports Science Association)

When practicing your moves with weighted objects, you risk developing *neuromuscular confusion* (you confuse the neuromuscular system), which creates:

• **Negative Transfer of Learning.** You will actually be a worse kicker after training with the weights than you were prior to training with the weights.

• **Incorrect Speed for Your Sport.** The weighted object might require you to practice at a slower or faster speed, or use different muscles than you use without the weight.

• **Possible Stress on Your Joints.** The weighted object might create bouncing or sudden tears of muscles or ligaments; for example, knee injuries or groin pulls.

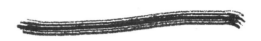

Training Tip

Power comes from strong muscles, not from repeated or specific movement. Remember, you must train with heavy loads to develop strength and explosiveness, so an ankle weight of a few pounds would not do the job. What you gain from lifting weights is *strength*, not specific martial arts skills. Good use of strength translates into power and good martial arts skills.

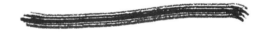

Biomechanical efficiency

Reaching biomechanical efficiency means that you have trained scientifically, within the confines of the laws of physics and biomechanics. You make every movement as mechanically efficient as possible and avoid wasted motion. The laws of physics and biomechanics have been verified through centuries of study and experimentation, and apply to all people at all times. Sometimes these laws work to your advantage, and sometimes they work against you. The trick is in knowing how to benefit from these laws. Having a basic understanding of elementary physics; that is, Newtonian physics, helps.

Newton's Laws of Motion

Newton's Laws of Motion are the backbone of the physics and biomechanical principles you will rely on to maximize your strength.

• **First Law:** An object in motion tends to stay in motion, and an object at rest tends to stay at rest, unless acted upon by some outside force. You must exert a force to set your body in motion from a state of rest, and you must exert a force to stop motion or change direction. If your opponent throws a punch, you need less force (strength) to evade his strike than to stop it. In fact, a slight reinforcement of his strike in the same direction, as you pivot to evade it, might throw him off balance. If you throw a strike that your opponent evades, when you miss, you must ensure that your body's balance remains above your foundation.

• **Second Law:** The acceleration of an object is directly proportional to the net force acting on the object, is in the direction of the net force, and is inversely proportional to the mass of the object. For example, when engaged in a grappling match against a heavy opponent, you must exert a greater force (more strength) moving him back or off of you than if he is lightweight. If you are lightweight, try to avoid getting into this situation.

• **Third Law:** To every action there is an equal and opposite reaction. When striking or blocking, you will experience an equal force against your striking or blocking weapon. Choose weapons that are structurally strong to avoid injury to your joints. For example, if you use the fleshy part of your forearm to block your opponent's strike, you will appear stronger than if you

block with your wrist.

In addition to Newton's Laws of Motion, there are many things you can do to tweak or fine-tune your body mechanics to decrease the risk of injury and increase the efficiency, speed, and power in your techniques. For example, if you throw a punch with your wrist bent, it can cause injury to your wrist. If you loop the punch on impact, the punch will lack power. Some people have a natural sense of correct biomechanics, but if you are not one of them, with conscious effort you can still learn these principles and benefit from them.

Training Exercise

Go out on the track and observe people running or jogging. Many people run with their feet turned slightly outward, which makes them lose mechanical efficiency. When running, the outside edges of your feet should be parallel, which will make you slightly pigeon toed. Pay attention to your foot placement next time you run.

Note that running up stairs or uphill is a good way to strengthen the quadriceps, but running down stairs or downhill is hard on the body, because it forces your joints to absorb three to four times the weight of your body. When running, each leg, upon impact, must support the entire weight of your body, and running down stairs or downhill places extra stress on your knees and lower legs. This impact force is a major contributor to injuries.

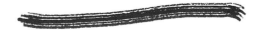

Applying the laws of physics and biomechanics to your training gives you a more effective power generation. In order to make these laws useful, you must understand several principles of motion:

Balance and Stability

Most of us know that the power in our strikes is practically worthless while we are in an unbalanced state, regardless of how muscularly strong we are. You are in constant motion when performing your techniques against an opponent, and several factors affect how well you maintain your balance when throwing a strike, taking a hit, or switching direction. The area of your base and your weight distribution directly affect your stability. A wide base is more stable than a narrow base, and a low center of gravity is more stable than a high center of gravity. It can also be said that a heavy person is more stable than a lightweight, mainly if you consider the fact that it requires more muscular strength to move a lot of weight than it does to move less weight.

- If you want to unbalance an opponent who maintains a wide and low stance, you appear stronger if you can first force him into a narrow stance or raise his center of gravity. If your opponent wants to unbalance you, you need to widen your stance and lower your center of gravity to better withstand the force he exerts against you.

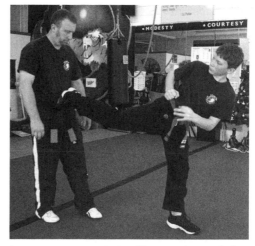

A narrow stance is ineffective for stability, and adds strength to your opponent's kick.

- In order to remain stable, your center of gravity must fall above the area of your base. For example, if you throw a spinning kick and fail to heed this principle, you will lose balance and, regardless of how muscularly strong you are, your kick will do little damage.

- The degree to which your center of gravity falls above the area of your foundation affects your balance. If your center of gravity falls near the edge of your foundation, you will be less stable in that direction than if it falls more toward the middle. If you throw a strike with your rear hand, and you allow your rear foot to come off the ground while extending your body forward, just a tiny re-enforcement of your strike, for example, by your opponent's parry, might throw you off balance. If you notice that your opponent is in the habit of being on one foot when striking, you can take advantage of it by parrying or pulling on his arm in the direction of his strike. This makes you appear stronger than you really are by using your opponent's lack of correct biomechanics against him.

• If your opponent weighs more than you, taking him off balance is more difficult than if he weighs less than you. Your relative build therefore affects your apparent or relative strength.

• If you need to accelerate from a standstill position, for example, when tackling your opponent, a center of gravity close to the edge of your base and in the direction of the movement helps set you in motion quicker. If you lower your head and arch your body forward when tackling your opponent, you will be faster and more explosive than if you tackle him from an upright stance, regardless of your muscular strength. On the other hand, if you need to run for distance, once past the initial acceleration, your body should take on a more upright position.

Distance and Timing

How you judge distance directly affects timing and, therefore, your strength and power. Normally, distance is constantly changing in the martial arts, but in general:

• If you are at the tip of your reach when striking, the only way you can strike through the target is by driving your body forward; in other words, by taking a step. If the target is located closer to your body, you decrease the risk of hyper-extending your joints or over-extending your center of gravity.

• If you time your strike to land when your opponent is stepping forward, you can appear stronger by relying on your opponent's momentum instead of your own.

Gravity and Inertia

Gravity is the force of attraction between the earth and your body. Inertia is the force that acts in the direction opposite of motion. Every time you move, you must overcome gravity or inertia in some way.

• Overcoming gravity and inertia requires muscular strength, and is especially prevalent in techniques that require an upward motion away from the earth's center of mass; for example, when performing a jump kick. Getting up from the ground when your opponent has taken you down is another example. The more you weigh, the more strength is required to counter gravity and inertia.

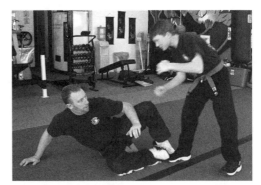

Getting up from a fall requires strength, because you must overcome the forces of gravity and inertia.

• Less obvious are moves that are parallel with the earth's center of mass, for example, when taking a step forward. However, raising your foot off the ground requires strength, and keeping your guard from sagging requires strength. Kicking downward, as in a stomp, or lowering your weight when striking your opponent makes you appear stronger than you are through the aid of gravity.

• When jumping, the power of your jump and the height you achieve is proportional to the angle between your upper and lower leg. A low bend in the knees prior to jumping creates a more explosive kick and therefore more apparent strength.

Gripping and Poking

Your gripping strength is along your power fingers, which activate your power muscles. Contrary to popular belief, your power fingers are not your bigger fingers, but the last two digits (little finger and ring finger). These are used for lifting or pulling, for crushing, or for any gross motor skills that require a lot of strength.

• When gripping your opponent to keep him from escaping, your power should be focused along your power fingers. The same is true when gripping a pull-up bar: Your thumb, which is not a power finger, should grip over the top the bar in the same direction as the fingers to avoid splitting the strength of your power fingers.

• Your guiding fingers are your first two digits (index finger and middle finger), and your thumb. These help guide and support the movement of your power fingers, and are used for activities requiring fine motor skills, such as precision when poking your opponent in the eye in a self-defense scenario. Your thumb is also used along with your index finger for fine motor skills, such as pinching specific nerve centers.

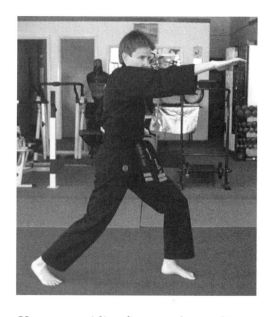

Use your guiding fingers when poking precision targets.

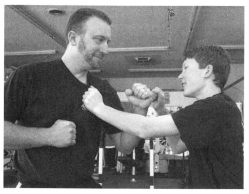

A crushing grip to a bigger opponent's chest muscle could get you his instant attention, and requires good gripping strength.

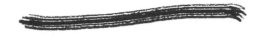

Gripping and Guiding Strength when Wielding a Weapon

When gripping and wielding a weapon, first look at the primary purpose of the weapon. If it is a club, you probably want to focus your grip on your power fingers. Note that I am saying *probably*, not always, as there are other factors to consider, for example, how to place your fingers on the weapon to avoid exposing them as targets. If it is a smaller weapon that needs a lot of manipulation, such as a knife or nunchaku, you might need to focus more on your guiding fingers.

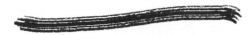

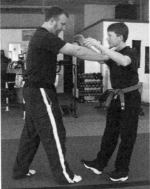

Failing to maintain your line of power (above) makes you lose balance when pushed. A good stance gives the smaller person a strength advantage (below).

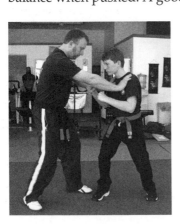

Leverage and Torque

When lifting a heavy object, such as your opponent or a rock you intend to throw at your opponent, you have more apparent strength if you keep the object as close to your center of gravity as possible. For example, lifting with your arms extended away from your body requires greater strength than lifting with your arms close to your body.

• When getting ready to lift, bring the weight close to your body, or bring your body close to the weight. The farther away the weight is from your body, the greater the torque. Torque = applied force X lever arm, and when the weight is far away, the lever arm is longer and more force is required to lift the weight. Biomechanics help you determine the correct distance from your body at which you should work a technique. Sometimes, a long lever arm can help you achieve strength, and other times, for example, when a weight is applied to the lever, a long arm can make you lose strength or strength efficiency.

• Your apparent strength relates to your line of power. In general, it can be said that you are strongest in the direction in which your stance is the widest, and an incorrect stance gives you a point of weakness in your line of power. For example, if you are in a horse stance, your line of power is to the side, and your point of weakness is straight ahead; you can easily be unbalanced in this direction. If you stand with one foot forward and one foot back, your line of power has shifted and is straight ahead, and unbalancing you is more difficult. Your line of power should always be in the direction of your work. If you are lifting a weight from left to right, you appear stronger if you pivot your legs along with your body and turn your line of power with the weight, than if you pivot your upper body or arms only.

• If you stretch your arms straight ahead from a neutral stance, and a weight is applied to your hands, you will have difficulty keeping your arms level or maintaining balance. If you switch to a one-foot forward one-foot back stance, your line of power has changed and you will be stronger and retain balance easier against a downward force on your outstretched hands.

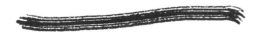

Leverage Tip

To gain an apparent strength advantage, keep your strength along your centerline. This is especially useful when lifting or working with only one side of your body. When lifting, or when being pulled or yanked, bracing yourself against any surface (hand on knee, hand against wall, etc.) gives you more apparent strength.

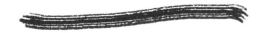

Mass and Momentum

Momentum, which is a combination of your weight and your motion, is one of the more important elements when determining your relative strength. In general, a heavy person has more natural strength than a lightweight, even if he is untrained in weight lifting. The more you can use your body weight, the stronger you appear.

• To maximize your apparent strength, use hip rotation or a step forward when throwing a strike, or use your weight against your opponent's weaker anatomy, such as his joints, in a grappling match.

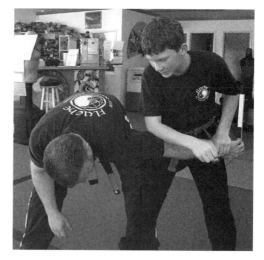

Weight combined with motion can give a smaller person the strength advantage, especially if used against an anatomically weak target, such as your opponent's joint.

• Although your mass (weight) is important, you must also have the strength to move that weight, because without motion there is no momentum. In general, weight and size benefit you in the martial arts, but there is a point at which your weight and size become cumbersome. If you are a large or heavy fighter, having good muscular strength helps you move your weight faster, which results in speed and acceleration, which results in power.

• Once you are in motion, coming to a sudden stop means that you must overcome momentum and inertia. One of the best ways to do this is by spreading your weight and lowering your center of gravity. If your opponent is tackling you, keep him from taking you down through this same principle. Spreading your weight and lowering your center of gravity make you appear stronger than you really are.

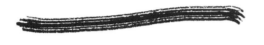

Training Tip

A strong strike requires a strong midsection and coordination between the upper and lower body. Over-extension results in balance or power loss. Practice balance and power for punching by throwing a weighted object, such as a 10-pound rock or medicine ball, while focusing on keeping your center of gravity above your foundation. Do not over-extend your body by leaning into the throw or raising your rear foot off the ground. If you add a trunk twist as you would when throwing a strike, you will notice how a strong midsection gives you more power.

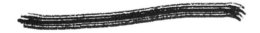

Work and Energy

When you get to wrestling or close range, the heavier fighter almost always has an advantage, and the lightweight has to expend a great deal of energy manipulating the bigger fighter's mass.

• When fighting at striking or kicking range, it is mostly your own body you are concerned with manipulating, and a lighter weight body is easier to move. When at grappling range, you must manipulate your opponent's body as well as your own, so a great deal of strength is needed, especially if he is heavy and trying to counter your efforts.

• Drawing your arm to the rear prior to throwing a strike places your arm behind your center of gravity, requires your arm to "catch up" with the rotation of your body, and wastes energy. You appear stronger if you keep your elbow in front of your body and let the strike originate in your body, not in your arm.

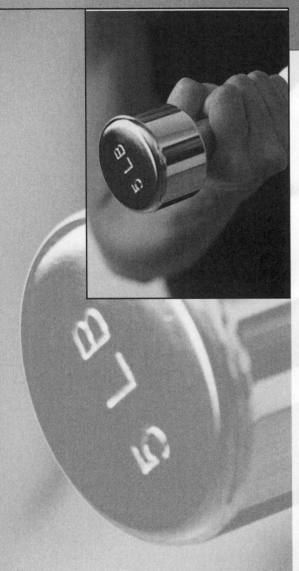

Understanding the Concepts

In this section:

- Acceleration
- Breathing
- Flexibility
- Intensity
- Machines or free weights
- Mechanics and momentum
- Midsection
- Multiple muscle groups
- Muscle mass and strength
- Muscular endurance
- Muscular failure
- Negatives
- Opposing pairs
- Over-training
- Progressive overload
- Range of motion
- Recovery time
- Repeated submaximal efforts
- Specificity
- Tensing
- Variation

Understanding the Concepts

We have now identified and discussed the importance of strength – muscle, bone, and joint anatomy – and the use of physics and biomechanical methods to help improve strength through correct movement of the body. Before learning how to build your strength using weight machines, free weights, and bodyweight exercises, I suggest you take a moment and review the concepts.

Acceleration

Muscular strength in the martial arts can be thought of as force development, or the ability to exert maximal force in a short duration of time, which translates into sudden acceleration against resistance. According to this definition, muscular strength is not the same as muscular endurance, which requires a sustained effort at less than maximal force.

You can train muscular strength and acceleration either by executing a "sprint" of the weight at the beginning of the repetition, or by pausing in mid-range. For example, if doing the bench press, grab the barbell and lift the weight to full range in one explosive move. To ensure acceleration and not just "fast lifting," the speed at the end of the concentric phase should be faster than at the beginning, while using correct form throughout the lift. You can also lift the weight to mid-range of the concentric phase, pause for a second, and then restart the lift against the resistance while accelerating the weight. Make sure you lower the weight with control.

By exerting brief maximal efforts, you improve muscular coordination. I recommend acquiring a good background on weight lifting technique first, prior to trying to accelerate the weight. But acceleration can add variety and help you achieve an edge when you are a few months into your weight lifting program.

Breathing

Correct breathing technique helps you maximize performance in weight lifting and sports in general. Exhale on the positive phase and inhale on the negative phase of the lift. Think of breathing as your *kiais* in karate. Avoid holding your breath through any part of the lift. Holding your breath can result in elevated pressure in the heart and abdomen, and can deprive the brain of oxygen. However, telling you to exhale is not the same as saying that your lungs should be like a limp garbage bag where all air escapes at once. For example, when you strike an opponent in the martial arts, you *kiai* and exhale. You increase power by tightening the abdomen (and your striking muscles) and exhaling in a short grunt. The same concept is used in weight lifting.

"Working with weights, the technique that should be used when doing any type of pushing movement, is to exhale as you thrust and inhale during the negative part of the movement. With pulling exercises, you do the opposite: exhale on the pull. Just remember to exhale on the exertion, pushing all your breath out from deep down, much like in karate when you go to strike an opponent. But anytime you're going to have to spend a lot of energy, anytime you have to grunt to complete the movement -- the breathing technique must be correct." (Lee Haney, former Mr. Universe and Mr. Olympia, www.viewzone.com)

Flexibility

When lifting weights, we are concerned primarily with building stronger muscles, and not with becoming more flexible. But we can often benefit in one area while working another. The process of building muscular strength helps you increase your flexibility by working your muscles through their full range of motion. Full range of motion encourages blood flow to the muscle, and helps you achieve control of your muscular power.

Lift for range, not for speed; do not simply try to get through the routine. We often cheat because we want to get as much done as possible in the shortest amount of time. A good way to learn how to benefit from full range of motion is by doing the weight lifting routine without any weight or resistance at first, while paying attention to how far you can stretch the muscle on both the positive and negative phase. Next, do the exercise with resistance. Finally, repeat the exercise one more time without resistance to get an additional stretch and help reinforce muscle memory.

Next time you lift weights, try pushing the weight a little farther than you normally would. For example, when doing the pushup, imagine pushing your shoulder blades higher than the rest of your back on the positive phase to help you stretch your arms and shoulders. Or when doing the seated row, pull your elbows as far back as you can and squeeze your trapezius muscle at the center of your back. Work through full range of motion on the negative phase as well.

Goal oriented training

You achieve maximum results by knowing your roadmap. Some planning is therefore necessary before you arrive at the gym. First, write a one-sentence description of your goal. Your description should be specific. A statement such as, "to become stronger," tells you little about the value of your goal. "To build leg strength for 15 minutes of continuous heavy bag kicking," is more specific, especially if you have noticed that a kicking workout exhausts you while your peers are moving ahead.

Your next step involves specifying the exercises. If you are looking at leg endurance, a 20-minute run uphill might be a good goal to strive for, followed by work on the leg press and hamstring curl machines. Continue your program 3 days a week for 2-3 weeks and make note of your achievements. You might need to tweak the program to include more variety or to work specific muscle groups.

The more aware you are of your goal, the easier it is to build a successful strength program. Set goals that are not too difficult, and that you can expect to achieve in 1-2 months. A week prior to reaching your goal, start planning your next goal, which could either be a tougher program than the one you are currently working on, or a goal for an entirely different muscle group.

Intensity

How much strength you gain is directly proportional to how hard you work and the weight of the loads you lift. So, yes, the no pain no gain principle is true. If you don't put anything in, you won't get anything out. Building strength takes work. For maximum gain, work multi-joint exercises, such as squats, presses, and rows at high intensity. In other words, lift heavy loads through relatively few repetitions, 6-10 repetitions per set are recommended. If you can do more than 8 reps, it is time to increase the load. Yes, you might feel cocky if you pump out 20 reps at fast speed, but for the purpose of building muscle and strength, that is not the best way.

Rest for 2-3 minutes between sets. Although shorter rest periods are beneficial when working on muscular endurance, they don't allow adequate recovery time for maximum hypertrophy (growth of muscle). Longer rest periods allow you to use greater resistance in your next set before fatiguing the muscle. If you want to increase the intensity, you can work single-joint exercises (also known as isolation exercises, because they isolate the muscle group and involve movement around only one joint), such as leg extensions and leg curls, and increase the number of repetitions while decreasing the rest period.

Machines or free weights

As long as you work your muscles to fatigue, you will realize strength gains regardless of whether you use machines or free weights. Although machines are generally safer and easier to use, they also tend to limit the movement to one specific muscle group. The use of free weights is often beneficial in sport specific training, because free weights have greater capacity for improving functional strength; that is, the type of strength you need for the performance of your sport. Free weight exercises involve motion around several joints simultaneously and demand greater tensing of the muscles to overcome instability. However, when lifting heavy free weights, you need a spotter to help you avoid injury.

Whether you choose machines or free weights may depend mostly on what is available. If you don't have access to a gym membership, free weights are relatively inexpensive and can be accumulated over time and be stored in your basement or garage for easy access at home.

Mechanics and momentum

To gain maximum benefit from weight training, the muscles must work the entire time. The movement of the weight over a distance should be the result of muscular effort. Use of momentum is counter-productive, since it results in the tendency for the weight to continue on its own over a certain distance and, therefore, deprives the muscles of continuous work. In other words, muscular tension is used to set the weight in motion, but not to keep it in motion. You use momentum when you "throw" the weight into position, rather than lifting at a controlled pace. Although this might make you feel as though you can pack on the pounds, you are really just cheating yourself out of an opportunity to build strength.

The use of momentum also increases the risk of injury, because you are not using proper form; for example, you might be arching your back when doing a biceps curl. It is also important to use proper mechanics when lowering the weight during the eccentric phase of the lift. If you let the weight drop with the aid of gravity, not only are you cheating yourself out of the benefits of the eccentric phase, you must also use your joints to stop the motion of the weight suddenly and, therefore, risk injury to your joints.

Eliminate momentum by pausing a second or two at the most difficult part of the lift. For example, when doing pushups, pause for one second an inch above the floor. Or when doing pull-ups, pause for one second a few inches below the bar. Then lift yourself higher until your chin is above the bar. Next time you go to the gym, take a few minutes and observe the rest of the clientele. Can you spot the lifters who use momentum instead of controlled technique?

Midsection

The midsection may be the most important muscle group, because virtually every move you make involves the midsection to some degree. You use the midsection when you kick, punch, throw, and wield a martial arts weapon. Many of us are not aware of the practical benefits of a strong midsection, and are more interested in the impressive looks of a well-developed six-pack. But remember that looks and strength don't necessarily coincide. In other words, it is not necessary to have a well-defined six-pack in order to have functional strength in the midsection. Muscles show best when the body is lean. But since we tend to pack on extra fat around the midsection even if we are not fat in general, it takes a very lean diet to give you a visible six-pack. Your primary goal should therefore be to have a strong midsection, regardless of whether or not that strength is visible.

Make an effort to work the abs every time you go the gym. It is generally recommended that you do ab work at the end of your session, so that you don't risk fatiguing your abs early and limiting the amount of work your larger muscle groups can do. However, if you find that you ignore

working the abs because you are tired or bored by the time you get to the end of your session, I recommend doing ab work first to ensure that it gets done. You can work the entire midsection – the lower abs, obliques, and upper abs – in 5-10 minutes.

Multiple muscle groups

Sports seldom, if ever, use only one muscle group at a time. Working the muscles in isolation is therefore not specific to most sports. Exercises that target multiple muscle groups are recommended over exercises that isolate the muscles. For example, bodyweight exercises, such as squats and pushups, are excellent choices, while weight machine exercises, such as leg extensions, normally limit the movement to only one muscle group at a time. Also, exercises that target multiple muscle groups more closely simulate the strength needed for the sport you are engaged in. No sport I can think of uses the muscles in isolation.

Start by looking at the body as a unit and not as an amalgamation of separate muscles. In general, exercise the muscle groups from largest to smallest. For example:

- Hips, butt, upper legs
- Lower legs
- Upper torso
- Arms
- Abdomen and lower back
- Neck

If you exercise the smaller muscles first, you risk fatiguing those muscles and the larger muscles cannot benefit maximally. However, some discretion is necessary. For example, if you have a tendency to slack on the abdominals, lower back, and neck, you might want to work these muscle groups prior to the rest of your body.

Muscle mass and strength

How bulky your muscles are is not necessarily an indication of your strength. Many factors must be considered; for example, bone length, muscle-to-tendon ratio, tendon insertion points, muscle cross-sectional area, neurological efficiency, and testosterone level. It is therefore not possible to simply look at another person and determine whether or not he is strong. Women, for example, who have less testosterone and, therefore, less ability to develop visible muscular growth, can still have considerable muscular strength without being bulky. To maximize strength, it is recommended that you lift heavy weights of approximately 90% of your 1-repetition maximum, that you do no more than 8 reps per set, and that you rest 2-3 minutes (sometimes as long as 4 minutes) between sets.

Muscular endurance

Muscular endurance is the muscles' ability to maintain contractile force over time. When training for endurance, your aim is to keep going for a long time, regardless of whether or not the force output is great. When training for endurance, more repetitions with slightly lower loads should be used. Do a minimum of 12 reps, but aim for around 15-20. In some cases, you might want to increase the number to 50 or even 100 repetitions per set. I do this frequently in pushups and dumbbell punching exercises, which I have found to be beneficial for developing upper body

muscular endurance.

Note: Some people are under the misconception that a high number of reps with very light resistance is the best way to build muscular endurance. But remember that the workout must still be challenging in order to benefit you. For example, doing 200 biceps curls with 3-pound dumbbells does not give you enough weight to present a challenging workout.

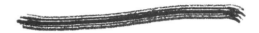

Muscular Endurance Test

Athletes with mainly slow-twitch muscle fibers can develop muscular endurance easier than athletes with mainly fast-twitch fibers. If you want to get an idea of how you rank, you can do an endurance test. First, find out what your 1-repetition maximum is in a given exercise, such as the bench press. Then lower the weight to around 80 percent of your 1-rep max, and do as many reps as you can. If you can do more than 15 reps at 80 percent, it is likely that you have predominantly slow-twitch fibers, which lend themselves to muscular endurance training. If you can only do 5-8 reps at 80 percent, it is likely that you have predominantly fast-twitch fibers, which lend themselves to muscular strength training.

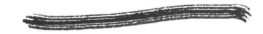

Muscular failure

It is not necessary to train your muscles to failure in order to realize results. Also, many people think they are training to failure, when they are really quitting because it hurts too much and not because they are unable to do one more repetition.

However, training to failure every so often might serve as a gauge to let you know what you are capable of. It tells you if you are using weights that are too light, or if you are doing too few reps to realize growth. For example, if you can do 22 reps with a specified weight before experiencing muscle failure, and you normally do only 11 reps before you think it starts to hurt and give in, you are way below your capability and must either increase the weight or increase the reps. If you can do that many reps, I recommend that you increase the weight. Be aware that if you do the muscle failure test at an inappropriate time, for example, when you are not feeling well or when you have over-trained, you will not gain a true measure of what you are capable of doing.

Muscular strength

Muscular strength is the muscles' ability to generate great amounts of force in a short period of time. Strength or power training is therefore high intensity for brief periods of time, and trains the muscles to create as much force as possible. Most martial arts are classified as power arts rather than endurance arts, although you must have muscular endurance as well if you want top performance.

Lifting for muscular strength normally involves 2-3 sets of 6-10 repetitions, with a load that is 80-90 percent of your 1-repetition maximum. Rests between sets should be slightly longer, with 2 minutes being a good rule of thumb. You can vary your training methods by increasing the load and decreasing the number of repetitions slightly, and resting for 3-4 minutes, or by decreasing the load and increasing the number of repetitions, and resting only as long as is necessary to perform the next set with good form.

Negatives

The negative or eccentric phase involves lowering the weight after having exerted your muscles through the positive or concentric phase. The negative phase is not a waste. In fact, significant strength building takes place during the negative phase as long as you use muscular control to lower the weight. For example, if you exhaust the muscles to failure during the positive phase, you can usually do a couple of negative reps and push past what you think is your limit. The negative phase is also extremely helpful when preparing for bodyweight exercises, such as pushups and pull-ups, if you lack the strength to do a full repetition through the positive phase. For example, when training to do pull-ups, start with five negatives; that is, start with your chin over the bar and lower yourself down slowly. This builds your strength, so that you eventually can do the full pull-up.

Along the same line as negative lifting are additional *forced reps* to failure. This requires a spotter to assist you. First, work to positive failure. Then:

• Use a spotter to help you through a few partial lifts to failure.

• Have a spotter remove part of the weight, and do a few more full lifts to failure.

• Have a spotter on stand-by, while you hold the weight steady in isometric contraction at mid-range of the positive phase to failure.

Opposing muscle groups

Remember, there are two sides to a joint, and you have muscles on both sides to allow the joint to flex (bend) and extend. When one muscle group contracts, the opposing muscle group lengthens. It is easy to over-train one side of your body while neglecting the opposite side; for example, to train your chest but not your back, or to train your biceps but not your triceps. The front of our body (quadriceps, abdomen, chest, biceps) tends to be stronger than the back (hamstrings, lower back, upper back, triceps). Some of this is because we use our frontal muscles more in every day activities, but also because we think a well-developed midsection or chest is more noticeable than a well-developed back, so we tend to work more on our frontal muscles.

The opposing muscle group is called the antagonistic muscle, and in order to avoid muscle imbalance and decrease the risk of injury, muscles should be trained in opposing pairs. I recommend designing a training schedule that alternates exercises for opposing muscle groups, so that when you have finished a set of leg extensions, for example, you do a set of hamstring curls.

Over-training

Yes, you can get too much of a good thing. Your training schedule must be sensible. Going to the gym every day, or spending 4-5 hours each time, can easily lead to over-training which is detrimental to the development of strength.

Over-training is defined as training that negatively affects your ability to perform your sport. This can happen when you are focusing on the wrong muscle group, when you are fatiguing your muscles

too much without giving them adequate time to rest, or when you are simply burned out mentally and don't desire to continue training. If this happens, you need to back off for a while until you can start making progress again.

Progressive overload

In order to develop strong muscles, you must overload the muscles and stimulate them to grow and handle the greater demands placed upon them. Muscles grow when they are challenged to grow. Without challenge, there is no growth. Or in practical terms, when an exercise is becoming easy, you must find a way to make it difficult. If you don't, you will stagnate; you may maintain your strength, but you will not improve. If you take a longer break or decrease the load, you will be unable to maintain your strength and your muscles will begin to atrophy from disuse. A proper strength-training program makes it appear as though you never arrive. Properly understood, this is your goal and should therefore not be discouraging. But it must be done with some forethought.

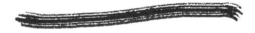

When Will I See Results?

If you train properly and with enough resistance, you can expect to see positive results in 3 weeks, and sometimes in as little as 10 days.

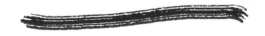

"The minimum resistance needed to obtain strength gains is 50 percent of the 1-RM (repetition maximum). However, to achieve enough overload, programs are designed to require sets with 70 to 80 percent of one's 1-RM." (www.survivaliq.com) For example, if your 1-repetition maximum is 150 pounds, this means that you should lift a weight that is at least 105 pounds (150 X .70 = 105) to get enough overload resistance.

Proper combination of four factors (repetitions, sets, specificity, and overload) leads to strength development. Generally, a good way to develop strength is to select a specific muscle group that you want to develop, find an exercise that requires the use of these muscles and use a moderate overload to stimulate the muscle group. Overload can be achieved, for example, by doing 3 sets of 8-12 repetitions. Do just one less repetition than what you can possibly do; that is, if you can do 11 repetitions but not 12, then do a set of only 10 repetitions. Although the experts differ somewhat on the number of repetitions and sets, this recommendation yields results.

There are many ways in which you can overload a muscle. But in order to benefit from overload, the muscle must be overloaded through its full range of motion. For example:

- Increase the resistance (the weight).

- Increase the number of repetitions per set, or keep the repetitions the same and increase the number of sets.

- Increase the speed with which you do the exercises. Remember to use good form. If you use momentum you will not realize any significant gain, and if your form is sloppy you risk injury.

- Decrease resting time between sets.

Range of motion

Training the muscles through full range of motion gives you the greatest strength benefit. Full range of motion eliminates the possibility of cheating by doing partial lifts, helps improve flexibility in the joints, and trains the muscle at every point of its range, which enables you to do that extra half-inch push when you need it in your martial arts training. Lift with controlled movement and avoid using momentum to achieve full range of motion.

However, there are some benefits to partial lifts. For example, partial lifts may help you reach a breakthrough by allowing you to lift heavier weights. Partial lifts can also decrease the risk of injury that typically happens at the weakest range of the joint, namely full range, and can help during injury rehabilitation.

Recovery time

Your muscles need time to recover after strenuous exercise. Recovery time is broken into two parts: days between training sessions, and minutes between specific exercises. For example, the muscles need approximately 48 hours of recovery time after a training session. This means that it is a bad idea to go to the gym and lift weights every day. Note that this does not apply to cardiovascular training. In other words, going for a run every day is not detrimental to your heart. However, be aware of the greater risk of over-use injuries, such as shin splints, if you never take a day off to rest from your cardio-training.

Your muscles also need time to recover

between sets within a training session. Normally 2-3 minutes of recovery time is recommended when lifting heavy loads for the purpose of building strength. Shorter recovery times are acceptable if working with lighter weights for the purpose of building muscular endurance. The intensity of your training should be dictated by the needs of your art, your health, possibly your age, and outside factors, such as your obligations to work and home.

Repeated submaximal efforts

The concept of repeated submaximal efforts relates to strength endurance, and is the ability to maintain a specific force repeatedly. Lifting weights repeatedly at slightly less than maximum resistance helps you build muscular endurance and a good general strength base prior to your sport specific development. The use of repeated submaximal efforts also helps you maintain good basic strength throughout life.

Specificity

In order to improve your martial arts skills through the use of strength training, the training exercise must be specific to the skill. Note that we are talking about martial arts *skills*, which means specific techniques. Do not confuse martial arts skills with being a "stronger fighter." In order to determine whether a strength training exercise is specific, it must pass four tests: muscle specificity, movement specificity, speed specificity, and resistance specificity.

• **The muscles** you wish to develop in the martial arts skill must be developed in the strength training exercise.

• **The movement** you wish to develop in the martial arts skill must be developed in the strength training exercise.

• **The particular speed** you wish to use in the martial arts skill must be developed in the strength training exercise.

• **The resistance** encountered in the martial arts skill must be the same as in the strength training exercise.

With the above in mind, it is easy to see that weight-training exercises generally do not mimic martial arts skills. The time you spend in the weight lifting gym should be used to improve strength; the time you spend in the martial arts training hall should be used to improve specific skills. However, improvement in your martial art is a by-product of strength. In order to gain an edge, you must do two things: Practice the art and develop stronger muscles, especially those muscles that are used the most in your particular art. A strong muscle does not give you a better martial arts technique, but a strong muscle can generate more force, which enables you to dominate your opponent, beat him to the punch, react faster to a threat, or last longer under pressure.

Specificity Principle

To improve your martial arts skills, you must practice your martial arts techniques. The same is true regarding specific components of strength. If you want stronger legs, doing 100 pushups a day will not help you. There is another way of looking at specificity: Just wanting to get in better shape or be the best that you can be is not specific enough. Wanting the strength to do 1 pull-up or 20 full pushups is more specific. Knowing *why* it is important to have the strength to do 1 pull-up or 20 pushups is even more specific. The training must also be specific to your individual tolerance to weight lifting, training stress, and outside obligations. Define your goals before starting your sport specific training program.

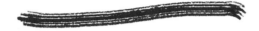

Sport specific exercises

Sport specific means that the exercises you do are specific to the sport you are trying to improve. For example, long distance running helps improve endurance for long distance running, but not necessarily for grappling or wrestling. In order to achieve maximum benefit from your training, first determine what exactly it is that you need. For example, if you need sprinting speed, you must train in sprints and not in long distance running. If you need explosiveness, you must train in plyometric exercises that include quick starts and stops of movement. If you need raw strength, you must train with heavier weights under controlled conditions.

After you have achieved a general strength base, design your training program for the purpose of enhancing your specific style of martial art. In order to do this, you must first analyze what type of strength is required for the successful performance of your art. Although good general strength throughout the body is required for all arts, your art might require more leg strength than upper body strength, or more muscular endurance strength than explosive strength. Once you have made this determination, you can design a program that will benefit

you the most with the least amount of wasted time and effort.

• If you are grappler or wrestler, leg strength is important because it allows you to push off, drive forward, and otherwise dominate your opponent at grappling range. To develop leg strength, do exercises such as squats, lunges, uphill hiking, and pushing drills against obstacles or barriers.

• If your art involves a lot of kicking, dynamic leg exercises might be a better choice than a standing squat or a low horse stance.

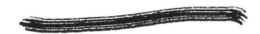

Is Cross-Training Beneficial?

Cross-training in different arts, or cross-training in different types of strength building exercises, may benefit you sometimes and work against you at other times, and depends on how sport or movement specific the cross-training is. Sport specific training is generally more effective than is cross-training at increasing performance for a particular sport, because it targets the specific muscle groups you are to use in your sport.

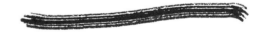

Uneven and unstable surfaces

When relying on bodyweight exercises, training on uneven or unstable surfaces forces you to exercise greater control over your muscular movement. In other words, you can't rely on a machine to keep the force properly lined up with the movement of the joint. This requires greater tensing of the muscles, which results in greater intensity workouts and, therefore, greater potential strength gains. Training on uneven or unstable surfaces, such as a grassy slope for pushups or a stability ball for ab exercises, should be done after you have mastered the basic movement on a flat surface and built a good general strength base. Be aware of greater risk of injury when training on uneven or unstable surfaces.

Tensing

In order for a muscle to contract, it must tense. Tensing helps you achieve greater strength gains and makes the exercise seem easier. This is especially noticeable in bodyweight exercises that require the movement of your body as opposed to movement of an outside object. It is easier to move your own bodyweight if your body is stiff than if it is limp like a sack of jelly. Try to pick up your child or dog when they don't want to get picked up, and you will know what I mean. Tense your muscles for a few seconds prior to doing a squat, pushup, or lift.

Variation

Strength training places continuous stress on the body part you are trying to develop. This requires adjustments in the routine to target slightly different muscle groups and avoid overuse injuries. When your muscles get used to a specific routine, they get comfortable and stop making gains. You must now make them uncomfortable again. Variation is important for several reasons: to keep you motivated and avoid boredom, to allow for strength progression even after your body has gotten used to a particular routine, to provide you with balance between upper and lower body, and to ensure that you work antagonistic muscle groups. If you alternate between lower and upper body exercises, you might also accomplish more in less time. For example, do a set of squats and then do a set of pushups.

You don't have to vary your routine every time you lift, but I recommend making some variation every 3-4 weeks. Write down a workout plan a few weeks ahead of time to help you stay on course and avoid getting sidetracked. "The human body will adapt to any exercise routine in approximately 4-6 weeks. If you do the same routine over and over, the body will adapt and become efficient at the movement. That's a good way to stall your progress." (Raphael Calzadilla, www.efitness.com)

Variation can come in several areas; for example, intensity, number of reps, amount of weight, days off between workouts, time between sets, and alternating upper and lower body exercises on the same day or on different days. Do not count the hours you spend at the gym. Doing something constructive is more important than training for long hours at a time. Try these variations:

• **Increase the intensity** each week, working faster through a particular set, cutting the time between sets, or adding additional weights.

• **Vary the workload** for the same types of exercises. For example, use lighter weights in the first set of the exercise, and heaver weights in the next set. Or do several sets, increasing the weight in 5-pound increments. Then work your way back down in 5-pound increments.

• **Do pyramids.** For example, sets of 2, 4, 6, 8, 6, 4, and 2 reps with constant resistance. Do some other exercise between each set, 10 pushups, for example. Or do pyramids, increasing the resistance while decreasing the reps. For example, 50 pounds X 10 reps, 60 pounds X 8 reps, 70 pounds X 6 reps, 80 pounds X 4 reps, 90 pounds X 2 reps, and 100 pounds X 1 rep.

• **Work according to time** rather than according to reps. For example, do a particular exercise for 30 seconds without counting reps. Rest for 30 seconds and repeat. I have found this to be helpful when working on muscular endurance training, such as dumbbell punching for a continuous 5-minute interval, going for 30 seconds on each of 10 different exercises. If you are just starting out, you might want to include a 15-second rest between each punching segment.

• **Vary the speed** with which you do the technique. Do a 3-count on the concentric move and a 1-count on the eccentric move. Reverse. Or try a full range explosive move with acceleration on the concentric phase.

• **Vary the sequence** of the different sets of exercises in your routine. Note that if one sequence seems more difficult than another, a reason might be because you are working the smaller muscle groups prior to working the larger muscle groups.

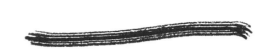

Variation in the Warm-Up Routine

Variation in warm-up can consist of shadowboxing one day, arm and leg rotations the next day, and a combination of pushups, situps, squats, and stretching the third day.

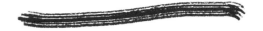

Machine and Free Weight Exercises

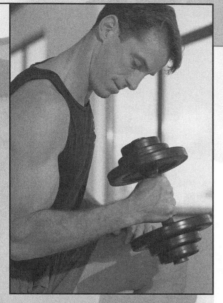

In this section:

- Leg press
- Barbell squat
- Leg extension
- Leg curl
- Hip abduction
- Hip abduction with resistance band
- Hip adduction
- Calf raise
- Bench press
- Seated press
- Bent arm fly
- Lateral raise
- Biceps curl
- Triceps extension
- Seated row
- Decline press
- Pull-up
- Dip

Machine and Free Weight Exercises

There has been much debate over whether it is better to use machines or free weights when training for strength. The bottom line is that intensity of training, and not machines or free weights, determine muscular growth. Greater intensity and resistance equal greater strength and muscular gain, regardless of how the resistance is provided. Whether you use machines or free weights may be a matter of what is most readily available. Let's do a quick machine/free weight comparison:

• Weight machines are generally more stable and safer than free weights, and you can lift heavy weights without a need for a spotter.

• Weight machines give you a greater variety of leg exercises and pulling movements, such as lat pull-downs and rows.

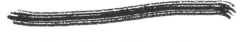

Functional Strength

When training on machines, you isolate the muscle groups. Since weight machines require no control of balance, they limit the transfer of functional strength. When it comes to sports, this type of training is a bit unrealistic, because virtually every sports movement requires several muscle groups to work together and not in isolation. I recommend using mainly free weights and bodyweight exercises, with the occasional weight machine exercise for variety.

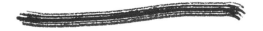

• Weight machines are usually set up at the gym so that you can quickly move from one to the other, and adjust the resistance in seconds.

• Free weights allow you to work your muscles in several planes and through greater ranges of motion.

• Free weights allow you to work under unstable conditions, requiring greater tensing and more muscular control.

• Free weights are relatively inexpensive and can be stacked in your home, if you can't afford a gym membership or a universal home gym.

• Free weights allow you to use different weights for the right and left sides of your body.

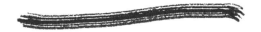

Asymmetrical Strength

Most people don't have symmetrical strength, so using uneven loads allows you to reach the greatest potential for each muscle group. For example, if you are right dominant, you will be stronger on your right side. If you allow your left side to determine the load, your right side cannot reach its greatest potential.

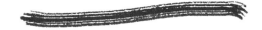

This chapter covers machine and free weight exercises for the lower and upper body. Remember that there are a large number of exercises and variations you can do to build your strength. Listing them all would be confusing and not time economical. I have therefore chosen to give you a fewer number of exercises that I have found to be beneficial in my own training. I encourage you to choose from these to form a basic and solid exercise program, and add your own variations if you have the need or desire.

Each exercise comes with a short description and lists the muscle(s) trained. Although many of the machine exercises are designed to train both of your legs or both of your arms together, it is often possible to work a leg or an arm singularly. This should be done if there is a significant strength difference between the left and right sides of your body.

When choosing exercises from this schedule, I recommend that you choose two exercises for each muscle group whenever possible; for example, one machine exercise and one free weight exercise. Supplement or vary your training with bodyweight exercises, as described in Chapter 7. Refer to Chapter 11 for abdominal exercises and to Chapter 10 for neck and grip exercises.

Training Tips

• Adjust the resistance or use heavy weights that allow you to do a maximum of 3 sets and 8 repetitions per exercise.

• Pause for one second at full contraction.

• Use controlled movements, and avoid dropping the weights with the aid of gravity or bouncing the weights against the weight stack.

• Do not lock your knees or elbows at full extension. Locking your joints eliminates the tension on the muscles and may hyper-extend the joint.

Leg Press
(Quadriceps, Hamstrings, Glutes)

Sit down and place your feet slightly wider than shoulder-width apart on the pad. The angle between your upper and lower leg should be about 90 degrees at the start of the movement. Press with your heels against the footpad until your legs are fully extended. Do not lock your knees.

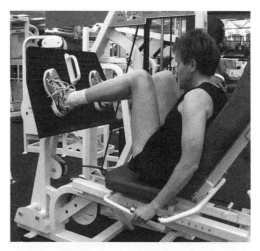

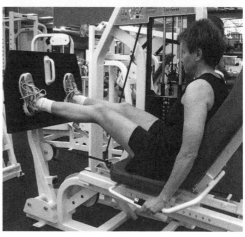

Barbell Squat
(Quadriceps, Hamstrings, Glutes)

Leg Extension
(Quadriceps)

Place a barbell across your shoulders (can also be done with dumbbells in your hands). Keep your feet about shoulder-width apart, and come down into the full squat position with your thighs parallel with the floor. Keep your back straight and your weight toward the heels of your feet. Press back up until your legs are straight.

Sit down with your feet extending past the roller pad. Extend your lower legs fully against the pad. There should be no movement in your upper legs. Keep your back firmly against the back pad, and avoid bouncing the weight against the weight stack.

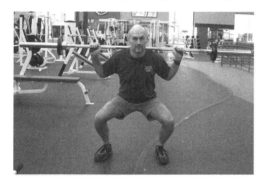

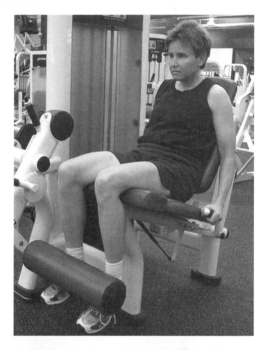

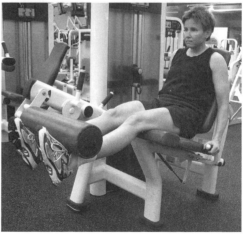

Leg Curl
(Hamstrings)

Sit down with your feet extending past the roller pad. Bend your legs until your heels are close to your buttocks. Extend your legs fully on the negative phase of the move, but be careful not to hyperextend your knees.

Hip Abduction
(Hip Abductors, Gluteus Medius)

Sit down and place your legs with the thigh pads slightly above and to the outside of your knees. Spread your legs by pushing against the pads. Keep your back against the backrest. Do not bend your upper body forward.

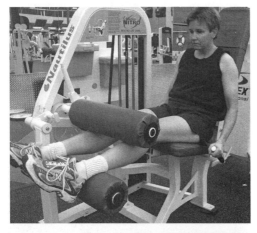
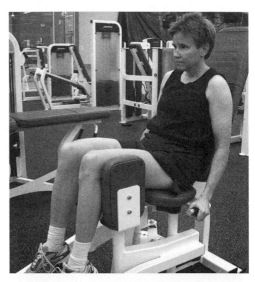
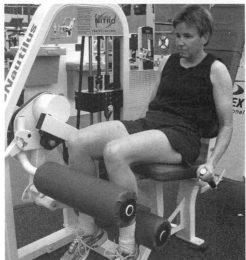
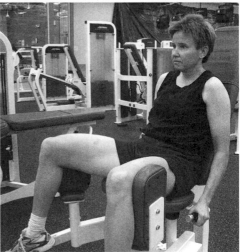

Hip Abduction with Resistance Band

(Hip Abductors, Gluteus Medius)

Stand on the resistance band with your feet close together. Grab one handle in each hand and stretch the band until there is tension. Walk to one side by stepping with your right foot first, hold the tension for at least one second, then step with your left foot. Repeat on the other side, or take ten steps to the right followed by ten steps to the left.

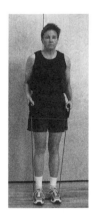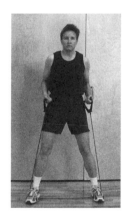

Hip Adduction

(Hip Adductors)

Sit down and place your legs with the thigh pads slightly above and to the inside of your knees. Bring your legs together by pressing against the pads. Keep your back against the back rest. Do not bend your upper body forward.

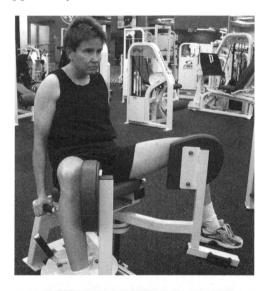

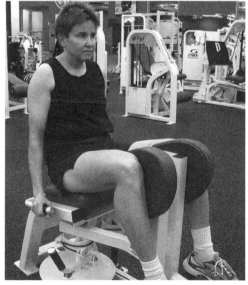

Calf Raise
(Calves)

Hold a dumbbell in your right hand and stand on a step or platform so that the heel of your right foot extends over the edge. Cross your left foot behind your right ankle. Raise up on the toes of your right foot, until your instep is in line with your shin. Keep your leg straight. Lower your heel as far as possible toward the floor. Repeat on the other side.

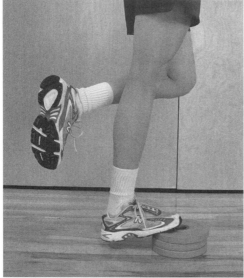

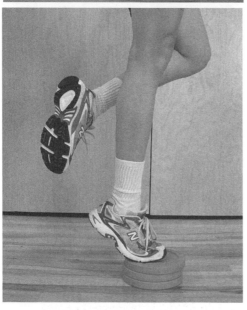

Bench Press
(Chest, Deltoids, Triceps)

Lie on your back on the bench with your feet flat on the floor. Grab the bar at slightly wider than shoulder-width, and press straight up from your chest. Lower the bar toward your chest. A very wide grip is not as effective because it reduces the range of motion.

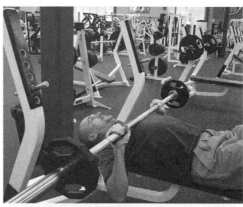

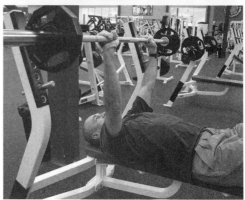

Seated Press
(Deltoids, Triceps)

Sit down with your feet flat on the floor. Grab the bar at shoulder-height with your hands slightly wider than shoulder-width apart. Press the bar up until your arms are straight.

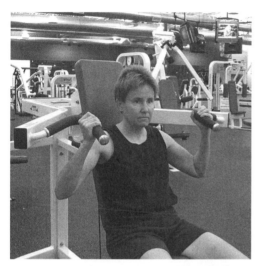

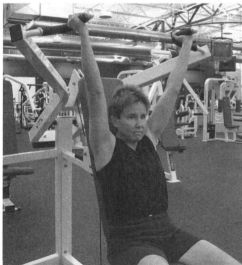

Bent Arm Fly
(Chest, Deltoids)

Lie on your back on a bench or exercise ball with your feet flat on the floor. Hold one dumbbell in each hand. Bend your arms and lift the weights until they are even with your chest. Turn your hands with your palms toward your feet. Bring the dumbbells together by lifting them up and toward your centerline. Your arms should still be bent at the completion of the technique.

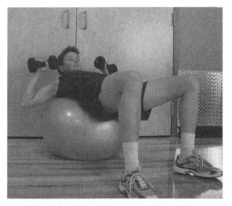

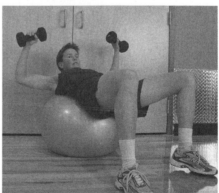

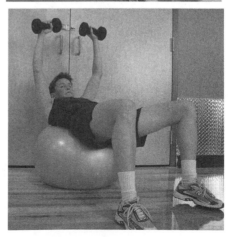

Lateral Raise
(Deltoids, Trapezius)

Stand with your feet shoulder-width apart and hold one dumbbell in each hand. Let your arms hang along the sides of your body, with the palms of your hands facing your legs. Raise the weights to your sides away from your body, until your arms extend straight out from your shoulders. Do not raise your shoulders.

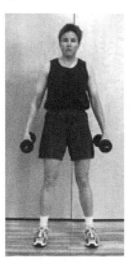

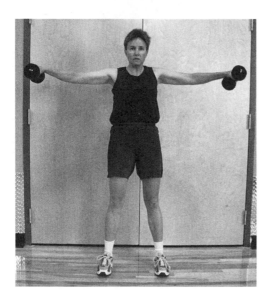

Biceps Curl
(Biceps, Forearms)

Stand with your feet about shoulder-width apart and grab one dumbbell in each hand, with the palms of your hands facing forward. Bend your arms and raise the weights toward your shoulders. Try the variation shown below: Stand with your feet together and start with your hands facing to the rear. Rotate your hands as you lift the weights, so that they are still facing to the rear at the completion of the technique.

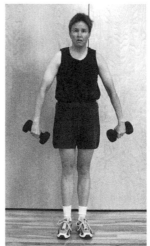
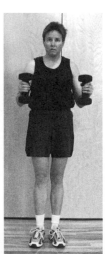

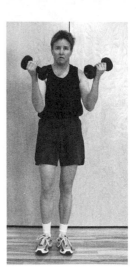

Triceps Extension
(Triceps)

Sit down with your feet on the floor, and place your upper arms against the pad. Grab the handles with your palms facing in. For maximum effect, keep your shoulders slightly lower than your elbows. Press away from you by straightening your arms. Do not allow your elbows to point to the sides.

Seated Row
(Lattissimus Dorsi, Biceps, Middle Trapezius)

Sit down with your feet on the floor or on the foot rests and grab the handles (some machines allow you to grab the handles with the palms of your hands facing either up or down). Pull the bar toward you. Do not swing your upper body to the rear, although some movement is permitted.

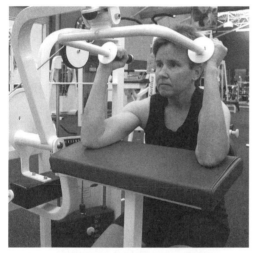

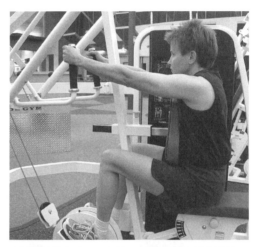

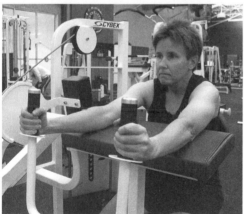

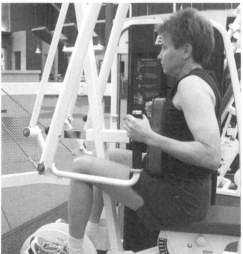

Decline Press
(Chest, Deltoid, Triceps)

Sit down and lean back against the backrest. Grab the handles with the palms of your hands facing forward. Push the handles away from you until your arms are extended. Bring your hands back to your chest.

Pull-Up
(Latissimus Dorsi, Biceps, Forearms)

Grab the pull-up bar and place your knees on the pad. Pull yourself up until your chin is above the bar. Vary your grip: wide, narrow, palms toward you, palms away from you, and palms in.

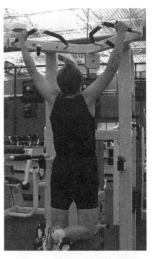

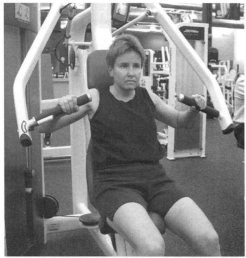

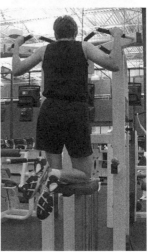

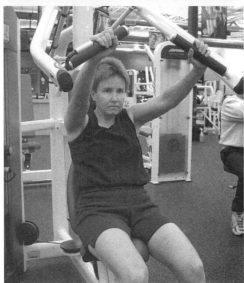

Dip
(Chest, Deltoids, Triceps)

Grab the handles with your palms facing in, and place your knees on the pad. Lower yourself down until your arms are bent 90 degrees. Press back up until your arms are extended.

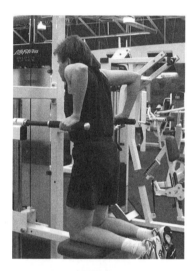

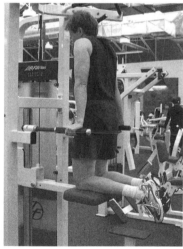

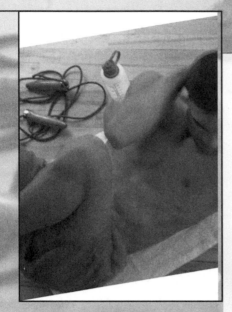

Bodyweight Exercises

In this section:

- The bodyweight challenge
- Progression without cheating
- The squat
- No-cheat half-squat
- One-legged squat
- Lunge
- Chair-stepping
- The pushup
- Inverted row
- The pull-up
- The situp
- Lower abs
- Obliques
- Upper abs

Bodyweight Exercises

There are many kinds of muscular strength exercises but for the purpose of building sport specific strength, I consider bodyweight training superior to regular weight lifting. Think about it: In just about every sport success depends on your ability to maneuver, lift, move, and manipulate your own body. You normally don't carry heavy weights in the martial arts, and most of what you do relates to your own bodyweight, or your weight in addition to a relatively light handheld weapon. Whether or not you can do a deadlift is therefore less relevant. Bodyweight training teaches you more than strength building; it teaches you strength building while moving.

When engaged in the martial arts, it is normally your entire body that must be moved, and not just an arm or a leg. You must therefore have a strong trunk along with strength in the extremities. Bodyweight exercises consist of squats, pushups, pull-ups, dips, situps, or anything else that requires the movement of your body as opposed to the movement of an external weight. Think about this: Although it may seem as essentially the same thing, sitting on a bench and pulling down on a resistance bar is not a substitute for the pull-up, because it is not your body you are moving. Likewise, lying on your back on a bench and doing a press is not a substitute for the pushup.

Strength is not valuable unless you can use it. Using your strength effectively in the martial arts requires good balance and control of your body while in motion. This is one reason I feel that bodyweight exercises are crucial; they give you the strength to move your body while maintaining balance.

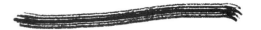

Relative Strength vs. Absolute Strength

Bench pressing 200 pounds is not as difficult for a 300-pound athlete as it is for a 100-pound athlete. In relative terms, the 100-pound athlete is therefore stronger. Whether this is useful or not depends on the situation. If it is a matter of moving your own bodyweight, relative strength is extremely useful. If it is a matter of defeating a much bigger opponent, absolute strength might mean more.

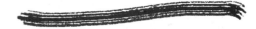

Benefits of combining machine and bodyweight exercises

Bodyweight exercises simulate your sport more closely than do weight machine exercises, and are useful for both the stand-up and grappling arts. Since the martial arts often require you to do the same move several times, you need endurance and the ability to move your body while maintaining balance in a variety of positions; for example, when throwing a kick or punch, or when pinning an opponent to the ground. All of this is developed through repetitive bodyweight exercises, such as pushups and squats.

A drawback is that there comes a time when your own bodyweight is not enough to provide the resistance needed to allow for muscular strength progress. Training with free weights and weight machines in combination with bodyweight exercises and endurance exercises, such as jumping rope and running, gives you a more complete workout that targets every muscle group.

Training Tip

It is good practice to train using a variety of equipment. This includes bodyweight exercises, free weights, and weight machines. If in doubt, remember that using sufficient resistance is more important than exactly what you use to provide that resistance.

The bodyweight challenge

Bodyweight exercises are difficult to do for many people, especially regarding the upper body. Pushups are hated, and pull-ups are so bad I'm going to make you do them just for spite! When starting out with bodyweight exercises, if you are unable to do a full pushup, pull-up, dip, or squat, there are many ways you can decrease the resistance without sacrificing good form. For example, if you have access to a gym, use a weight machine that has a counterweight specifically designed for giving you assistance. Or find something in the environment, such as a chair, tabletop, or hill. For example:

• If you are struggling with the pushup, do it on an incline first. Place your hands on a table or chair, or do a negative pushup, starting in the up position and slowly lowering yourself toward the floor. DO NOT do pushups on your knees. Knee pushups are almost worthless for building upper body strength.

• If you are struggling with the squat, place your hands on a tabletop to stabilize the technique and help yourself back up. DO NOT cheat by squatting only halfway.

Again, half-squats are nearly worthless for building lower body strength.

• If you are struggling with running, start by running on a slight incline downhill. DO NOT cheat by walking. Walking has its place in general conditioning, but if you want to build strength for the martial arts, you must push yourself past your comfort zone.

A Word about Cheating

As long as you are using proper form and full range of motion, you are not cheating when using an incline for the pushup or a tabletop for the squat to decrease the resistance. The same is not true for pushups on your knees or partial squats, which do not use proper form or full range of motion.

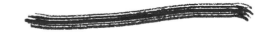

When doing assisted bodyweight exercises, try to limit the assistance to about 10-15 percent of your unaided attempt. If you need more assistance than this, you may want to build your general strength base first. In other words, the exercises should not be so easy that you can pump out 30 or 40 reps effortlessly. You must exert your muscular strength, or you won't see results.

The Bodyweight Challenge Pyramid

30 pushups, 30 squats, 30 situps
25 pushups, 25 squats, 25 situps
20 pushups, 20 squats, 20 situps
15 pushups, 15 squats, 15 situps
10 pushups, 10 squats, 10 situps
5 pushups, 5 squats, 5 situps

When you get down to the last 5, increase by 5, until you are back up to 30 for each exercise. This is a challenging workout that will whip you into great shape.

Progression without cheating

Although bodyweight exercises make it difficult to pack on the same amount of resistance you can achieve with machines or free weights, bodyweight exercises are not limited by the weight of your body. When the exercises become easy, you can increase the difficulty by elevating certain parts of your body, by working on uneven or unstable surfaces, or by doing the exercises on one leg or one hand. For example, elevate your feet when doing pushups, do one-legged squats, or run uphill. However, if you need a lot of resistance, you might need to resort to weights or a weighted vest.

Training Tip

When bodyweight exercises become easy, rather than picking up handheld weights, if possible, use a weighted vest. This allows you to preserve the basic exercise, without changing the move or inducing faulty muscle memory.

Let's look at progression in the bodyweight routine. First, you don't need to do a hundred pushups or squats every time you train. It is better to do 2 or 3 sets of 8 reps in the first couple of weeks, and then increase to 10 or 12 reps. When this becomes easy, increase the difficulty of the exercise and go back to the lower number of reps; for example, by doing pushups on a reverse incline or by wearing a weighted vest. You have now increased the resistance, which will help you build muscular strength without increasing the reps.

Next, add instability to increase the difficulty of the exercise. Any bodyweight exercise is by nature less stable than any machine exercise, but training on an uneven or slightly unstable surface, such as a grassy slope or a stability ball, forces you to tense your muscles even harder. More tensing translates into greater strength. *Caution: If using unstable surfaces, especially for lower body exercises, be careful so that you don't twist your ankles or lose your balance.* Make sure that you have a good general strength base first, before using exercises that require instability. Let's break down the bodyweight exercises in greater detail.

The squat

The squat has been termed "king of quad exercises." For lower body strength, the squat takes the prize, and a properly executed squat generally doesn't need more than your bodyweight to be effective. Squats are tough. They hurt. They are supposed to be tough and hurt. The problem is that most of us are too easy on ourselves. We claim to squat to the proper position, we claim to squat this incredible amount of weight, but we seldom work as hard as we think. In fact, we cheat shamelessly right in front of our instructor, hoping that he won't notice. And most of the time he doesn't, because he is either uneducated or inattentive. Train the squat without cheating and develop awesome lower body strength. Or quit when it starts to hurt. Or cheat. But remember, you are not cheating your instructor; you are cheating yourself. It is better to do a few bodyweight squats with proper form, than to do a hundred half-squats that don't build your legs. Start with your bodyweight and develop proper squatting form before adding additional weight.

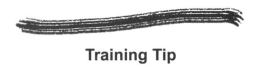

Training Tip

To squat without cheating, start by observing yourself in a mirror. The most common problem is that we don't squat low enough. Your thighs should be parallel with the floor. Grab a bo-staff and place it across your thighs. If it rolls off, you are not squatting low enough.

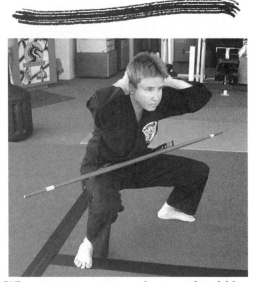

When you squat correctly, you should be able to balance a staff across your thighs.

The squat works the quadriceps, hamstrings, glutes, and calves to a lesser degree. The squat is a good lower body exercise, because it works more than one muscle group at a time. The squat, or the one-legged squat if you get this far, will help you develop good overall strength in your legs; it will help you develop legs that are strong enough to perform explosive jump kicks. If these are part of your martial art arsenal, the squat is a necessity. Good leg strength also gives you the ability to sprint away from an attacker on the street.

I will now exercise my bragging rights, just to let you know what can be achieved with training. I don't look overly impressive when it comes to muscular build; in fact, I look kind of average. Nobody would turn their head and comment on my build when I pass them on the street. But I hold a personal squatting record of 630 squats, which I reached as a result of being challenged to a squatting competition in 2003. I did 22 minutes of continuous squats, while the sweat was pouring off of me. I decided to quit when I got to 630, not because I was at the end of my rope (well, I admit, my legs were quivering a bit), but because I had outdone my closest competitor by 500, and I didn't see the point in continuing. I was able to walk up one flight of stairs immediately after finishing the contest, but my legs were twitching all night and I couldn't walk straight for six days!

But the squat is bad for the knees, you say. This is a common excuse, however, a properly executed squat is seldom bad for healthy knees. If you have a prior injury, you might possibly have a problem with the squat, and might have to substitute another quad exercise. Follow these squatting suggestions:

• Do the squat with the top of your thighs parallel with the floor.

- Keep your feet approximately shoulder-width apart, and your toes pointed slightly to the outside.

- Keep your back slightly arched, and your weight on your heels when lowering yourself down in the squat.

- Do not extend your knees forward of your toes.

- When coming back up, drive with your heels. Do not move your weight to the balls of your feet.

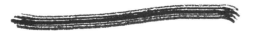

Training Tip

Prior to starting today's lower body strength training, hold the full squat position for 10-15 seconds to help you stretch and get comfortable with the exercise.

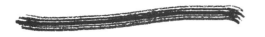

Are there any easier leg exercises than the squat? How about leg presses or leg extensions on weight machines? Remember, it is the intensity of training that determines your strength benefit, not whether the exercise is done on machines, with free weights, or using bodyweight only. However, bodyweight exercises and free weights are recommended over machines, because the instability factor forces you to use more muscular control. In addition, weight machines often develop only one muscle group at a time, so they are not as time-economical or as sport specific as bodyweight exercises. For example, the leg extension on a machine works only the quadriceps. The hamstring curl on a machine works only the hamstrings. The same is not true for the squat, which works the quadriceps, hamstrings, glutes, and calves together.

Squat variations include the half-squat (actually the *no-cheat* half squat), the one-legged squat, the lunge, and chair stepping.

Squat
(Quadriceps, Hamstrings, Glutes, Calves)

Squat until your thighs are parallel with the floor and your weight is slightly back on your heels. Do not extend your knees forward of your toes. Start with 2 sets, 8 reps.

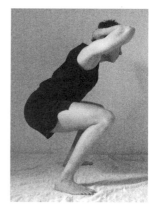

Correct: Weight on the heels, thighs parallel with the floor, and knees in proper position.

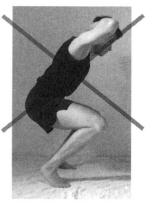

Incorrect: Weight on the balls of the feet, thighs not parallel with the floor, and knees extending too far forward.

No-Cheat Half-Squat
(Quadriceps, Hamstrings, Glutes, Calves)

Start with your feet about shoulder-width and a half apart and lower yourself toward one side, until that thigh is parallel with the floor. Do not extend your knee past your toes. Hold the down position for two seconds. Stand back up and repeat on the other side. Start with 2 sets, 8 reps.

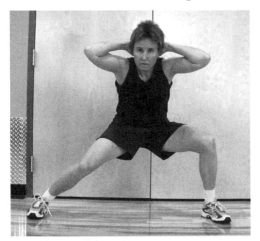

One-Legged Squat
(Quadriceps, Hamstrings, Glutes, Calves)

The one-legged squat involves balancing on one leg while coming down in the squatting position with your thigh parallel with the floor. You can keep your free leg in front of you or behind you. Most people find it more difficult to squat with your free leg in front. If you lack the strength to do the one-legged squat, use some assistance; for example, hold on to a tabletop, or sit on a chair and rock forward and up, then sit back down on the chair. Start with 2 sets, 3 reps.

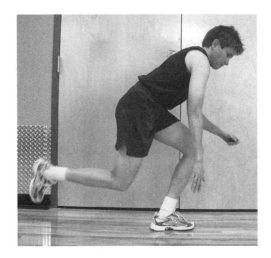

When starting with the one-legged squat with your free leg behind you and your upper body inclined slightly forward, attempt to go low enough that you can touch the fingertips of your vertically extended arm to the floor.

One-Legged Squat Training Tips

- When doing the one-legged squat with your free leg behind you, bend your upper body forward slightly to keep your balance. Do not get up on your toes. You can also reach your arms forward if it helps with balance, or reach down and pick something up from the ground to ensure you are going low enough.

- When doing the one-legged squat from sitting on a chair, first place one foot on the floor in front of you and do not move this foot. Keep this leg bent so that your thigh is parallel with the floor. Extend your other leg straight out. Rock forward on the chair until your butt comes off the seat. Continue into the one-legged squat position. Keep your weight toward the heel of your foot.

Lunge
(Quadriceps, Hamstrings, Glutes, Calves)

The lunge is a great exercise that, just like the squat, works the various muscle groups of the lower body. Lunges are also skill specific to martial arts. For example, we lunge in order to attack quickly and retreat quickly. Those engaged in fencing use the lunge as a fundamental move when advancing with the fencing foil. For the purpose of building lower body strength, the wider the lunge, the more effective it is. Bring your thigh parallel with the floor. Do not allow your knee to extend past your toes.

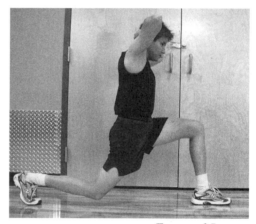

Forward Lunge

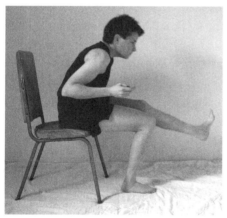

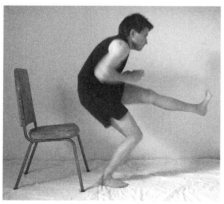

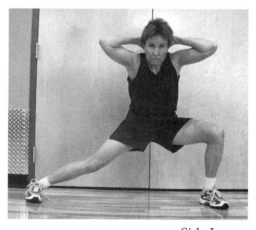

Side Lunge

Chair-Stepping

(Quadriceps, Hamstrings, Glutes, Calves)

Another way to strengthen the legs is by stepping up on a chair with one foot at a time. *Be aware that if you want to gain any benefit from this exercise, the stepping leg must do the work. Do not push off against the floor with your non-stepping foot.* Your thigh should be parallel with the floor at the beginning of the exercise. If this is too tough, start by stepping onto a lower object. Keep your upper body straight and your weight centered over the heel or middle of the stepping foot. Start with 2 sets, 5 reps.

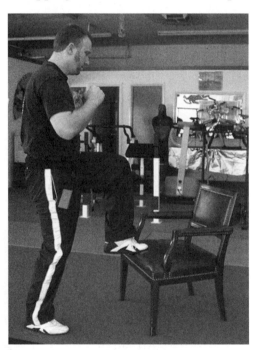

The Pushup

In my opinion, the pushup is one of the best bodyweight exercises for developing upper body strength. Pushups work the pectorals (chest), anterior deltoids (front of the shoulder), triceps (back of the upper arm), and the abs and lower back. The pushup requires strength in the back and midsection to keep your body from sagging. The pushup teaches you how to manipulate your own bodyweight before moving on to manipulating free weights or machines. The pushup is also time and space economical; you don't need any equipment to do it.

When doing the pushup, lower yourself until your upper arms are parallel with the floor, or until you are low enough to touch your nose to the floor or to the back of your partner's hand. You can do the pushup with your hands in a variety of positions to target slightly different muscle groups: wide, normal, narrow, or turned sideways or toward you. You can also place one hand higher than the other or, if you are very strong, do one-handed pushups.

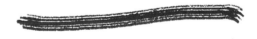

Training Tip

When starting out with pushups, do as many as you can and pay attention to which part of your body seems to limit the number of pushups you can do. This will help you determine where your weakness is. For example, if you can't push up from the floor, your pectorals are weak. If your body sags in the middle, your abs or back are weak and need additional strengthening.

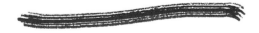

But if the pushup is so beneficial, why is it such a hated and grueling exercise? Why is it often used as punishment in the martial arts and the military? Personally, I love the pushup. When I'm at the gym, I go alone, I don't associate with anybody, and I follow a strict program. But I still observe other people and lifting styles. I observe their physique and note who is dedicated and who is not, who might be on supplements, legal or otherwise, and who is clean. Since I observe others so much, it is only natural to wonder if anybody ever notices me. Then, one day, I received a compliment that made me burst with pride. I was about to leave the gym after finishing my usual 320 pushups (not all at once, but interspersed with a 3-mile run, 200 ab exercises, 30 pull-ups, and a few sets on the weight machines), when this huge bodybuilder walked out and held the door open for me. Once outside, he asked, "Are you a drill sergeant?" Before I had answered, he continued, "You put the U.S. Marines to shame!" I knew then that somebody had noticed my routine. *Being unable to do pushups is not your fault; failing to do something about it is.* Make friends with the pushup. It is a great upper body strength exercise that also lets others know that you are dedicated in your training.

Pushup
(Pectorals, Anterior Deltoids, Triceps)

Keep your legs and back straight. Tighten your abs to hold in your midsection. There should be no sagging or bridging in your back. Keep your hands level with your armpits. Hands forward or to the rear of your armpits will make the pushup more difficult. Also try the hands wide or hands narrow positions. Start with 2 sets, 10 reps.

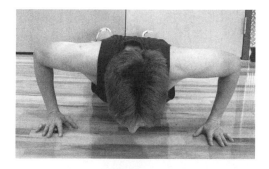

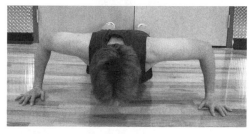

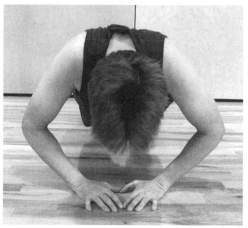

Inverted Row
(Upper Back)

After you have done a set of pushups, do a set of inverted rows using your bodyweight to work the antagonistic muscle. Lower the pull-up bar to about hip level. Place your feet on a chair, grab the bar, and hang in the horizontal position. Pull yourself up until your chest is touching the bar. If you are unable to do this, start with your feet on the floor instead of on a chair and raise the bar a bit higher, so that you are pulling on an incline. Start with 2 sets, 5 reps.

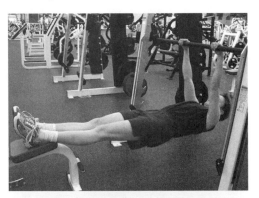

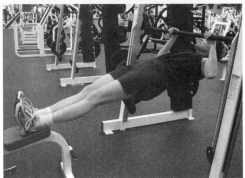

The Pull-up

The pull-up has you lifting a hundred percent of your bodyweight, and is the most difficult upper body strength exercise using your own bodyweight. The reason the pull-up is so difficult is because you must lift your entire body using only the smaller muscles of your upper body (remember, your biggest muscle is your butt). My opinion is that the pull-up is not a useful strength exercise for most people, until you have achieved a very good general strength base.

There are a number of ways you can do the pull-up: palms forward, wide or narrow grip, palms toward you (chin-up), or palms facing each other. Most people find the palms forward wide grip pull-up the most difficult, because your weight is not aligned with your centerline and you are using more of your upper back and lats than your biceps or centerline strength. The chin-up is normally considered the easiest.

Depending on the width of your grip, the pull-up works your back muscles slightly differently. When using the wide grip, place your hands about 6-8 inches wider than your shoulders. If your grip is much wider than this, you are depriving your muscles of full range of motion. After pulling yourself all the way up with your chin over the bar, slowly lower yourself down to the straight-arm position. Do not use gravity to drop your bodyweight back down. Using gravity not only defeats the benefits of the negative phase of the pull-up, you also risk injury to your joints. Note that when you reach the full down position, your feet should not be touching the floor and your arms should be straight. However, this does not mean that you should lock your elbows.

If you are not strong enough to do pull-ups, start with negative pull-ups, assisted pull-ups on a machine, or assisted partner pull-ups. Remember, the negative pull-up involves lowering yourself gradually until you are at the straight-arm hang position. Then let go, step back up on the chair, grab the pull-up bar with your arms flexed, and repeat.

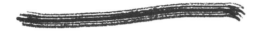

Exercise Tip

Contract your back muscles when doing the pull-up. Pushing your chest out slightly while pulling up might help remind you to contract your back muscles. You can also think of it as squeezing your shoulder blades together.

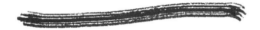

Pull-Up
(Trapezius, Latissimus Dorsi, Deltoids)

The pull-up can be done with the palms facing forward or toward you. It is then called a chin-up. Palms forward is the more difficult version, especially with your hands in the wide grip position. When pulling up, squeeze your trapezius muscle together at the center of your back. Your arms should be completely extended between reps, but do not lock your elbows. Start with 2 sets, 3 reps.

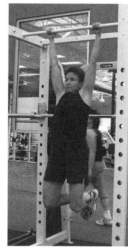

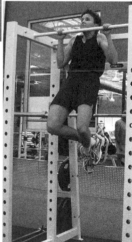

The Situp

Let's end this chapter on bodyweight exercises with an ab routine using only your bodyweight. Do the full routine with no break between sets and keep your head off the floor on all lower body ab exercises. Stretch when you are done. For more extensive information about ab work, refer to Chapter 11 on Abdominal Strength.

Mountain climbing, 20 reps each leg
Leg spread, 10 reps
Leg raise, 10 reps
Reverse crunch, 10 reps

Diagonal crunch, 10 reps each side
Side bend, 10 reps each side
Side V-up, 15 reps each side
Alternating reverse crunch, 15 reps

Crunches, 20 reps
Alternating diagonal crunch
    legs vertical, 15 reps each side
Straight crunch legs vertical, 10 reps
Sitting knee crunch, 15 reps

Lower Abs

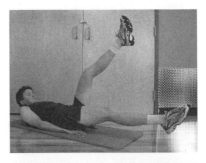

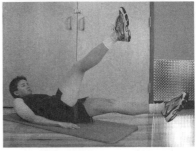

Mountain climbing, legs slightly bent 6 inches off the floor, alternate long stride. This is not a bicycle move!

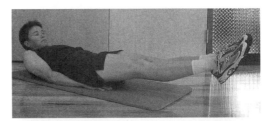

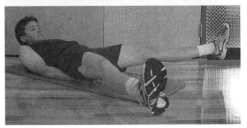

Leg spread, pause for a second at full spread position.

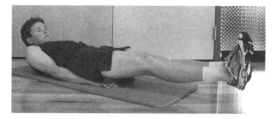

Obliques

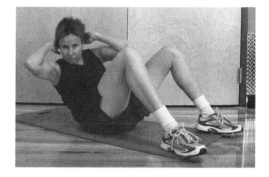

Diagonal crunch, left elbow to right knee, drop down to the middle, right elbow to left knee.

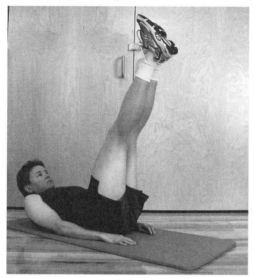

Leg raise, do not touch feet to the floor.

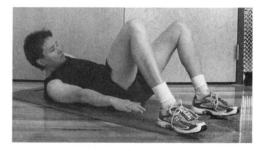

Side bend, reach with your hand toward your foot while crunching your side.

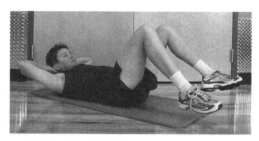

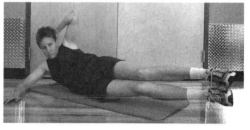

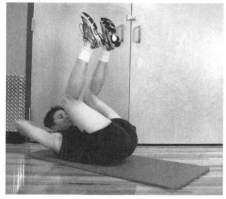

Reverse crunch, roll lower body toward upper body, lift hips off the floor.

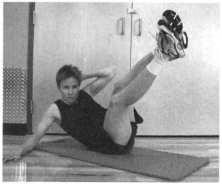

Side V-up, crunch upper and lower body, do not touch your feet to the floor.

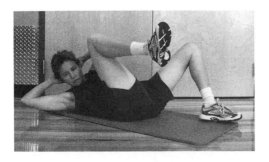

Alternating reverse crunch, right knee to
left elbow, alternate.

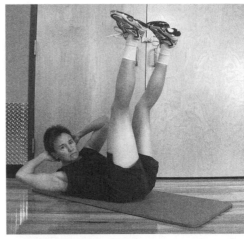

Upper Abs

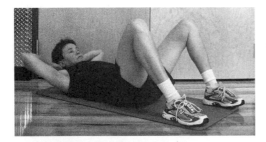

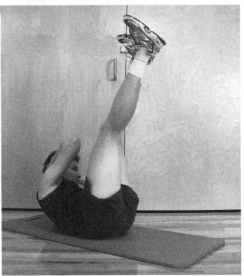

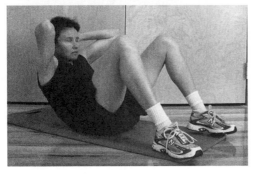

Crunch, bring upper body about 30
degrees off the floor.

Diagonal crunch, legs vertical, left elbow to
right knee, alternate.

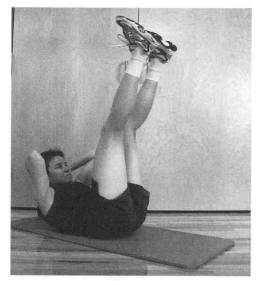

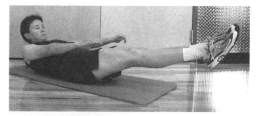

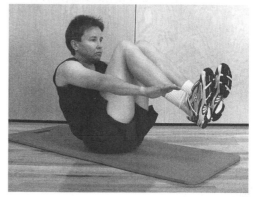

Sitting knee crunch, bring upper and lower body together.

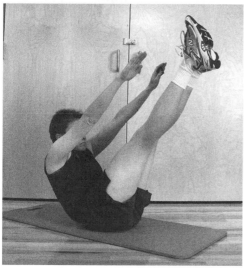

Straight crunch, legs vertical or at slight angle.

Building Your Strength Base

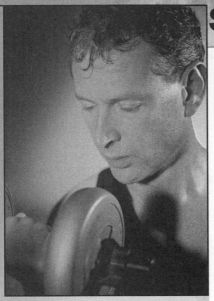

In this section:

- Muscular endurance

- Muscular strength

- Cardiovascular endurance

- Mobility/flexibility

- Rest and recovery

- Injury rehabilitation

- Circuit training

Building Your Strength Base

You have now received some instruction in using weight machines and bodyweight exercises, so you should have a basic idea of strength training. But to enhance your performance past the ordinary, you need to train sport specific skills and sport specific strength. First, you need a good general strength base to fall back on. General strength is a combination of muscular endurance, muscular strength, cardiovascular endurance, and mobility/flexibility. You also need a good understanding of rest, recovery, and injury rehabilitation.

Your general strength program includes all major muscle groups in the lower and upper body. It is recommended that you exercise the larger muscle groups prior to exercising the smaller muscle groups, in this order:

- Buttocks, hips, and legs
- Upper back and chest
- Arms
- Abdomen and lower back
- Neck

If you start with the smaller muscle groups, you risk not having enough energy left for giving the larger muscle groups their fair share of the workout. Personally, I am not a strict proponent of this principle. As you get to know your body better, you might find that you can have a more productive workout if you reverse or vary the order of some of the exercises.

You will gain greater benefit in general strength if you can set a program that is somewhat regular. Try to exercise at least three times per week and, if possible, evenly spaced; for example, Monday, Wednesday, and Friday. Disciplining yourself to participate in a general strength program with regularity helps you overcome the hurdle of exercising that so many of us feel.

Engage in the general strength program for about 6 weeks before getting into your sport specific training. You should see significant improvements in general strength in 2-3 weeks. A good general strength goal to shoot for is:

- 20 bodyweight squats with good form

- 10 full pushups with good form

- 30 situps with good form

- 1-mile run in 12 minutes

- No stiffness or soreness when moving your joints

These requirements should be achievable for just about everybody. If you have a prior injury, medical condition, or other limitation, make sure you check with your doctor and use good judgment when setting your general strength goal.

Muscular endurance

Muscular endurance is the muscle's ability to continue contracting and enduring a specific and steady intensity over a long period of time. Note that muscular endurance is not the same as *cardiovascular* endurance. Good muscular endurance enables you to hold a position or do repeated movements with the same muscle group without getting tired. An example is forms training at a specific intensity without slowing down, stopping, or regrouping. Another example is a sparring session where you throw a flurry of strikes and kicks, then slow down or move out of range to regroup, and come back with another flurry. If you have good muscular endurance and your opponent doesn't, you increase your chances of winning, because you can pick up the pace when he can't.

Muscular endurance is broken down into dynamic and static muscular endurance:

• **Dynamic muscular endurance** is the muscle's ability to contract and relax repeatedly. Throwing multiple strikes with the same arm without slowing down or lowering your guard is a demonstration of dynamic muscular endurance. Doing pushups until you experience muscle failure is a demonstration of dynamic muscular endurance.

• **Static muscular endurance** is the muscle's ability to hold the contraction for a period of time. Extending your leg in a sidekick and holding that kick is a demonstration of static muscular endurance.

Minimum General Strength Training Requirements

Muscular Endurance Training = 30 minutes, 3 times/week

Muscular Strength Training = 20 minutes, 2 times/week

Cardiovascular Training = 20 minutes, 3 times/week

Mobility/Flexibility Training = 10 minutes/day

If this seems like much just to reach a general strength base, keep in mind that you can combine many of the workouts. For example, stretch as warm-up and cool-down prior to and after your strength and endurance workouts. Some of the muscular strength and endurance requirements carry over into cardiovascular fitness. For example, running improves the muscular endurance of your lower body, while also improving your cardiovascular endurance. Swimming improves muscular endurance and flexibility in your shoulders. Your regular martial arts classes also count toward part of the general fitness requirement.

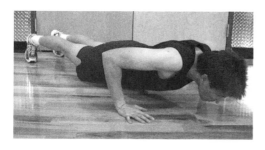

Holding a pushup two inches off the floor in the flexed arm position is a demonstration of static muscular endurance.

Good muscular endurance allows you to outlast your opponent. It allows you to throw more punches with greater speed, or continue pressing or dominating your opponent in free sparring or grappling. You might feel the greatest need for muscular endurance when under pressure to perform, for example, when in a sparring match that requires barrages of strikes and kicks to keep your opponent at bay. In the weight lifting gym, I have found that moving quickly from one exercise to the next, without giving the muscles a lot of time to recover, is a great test of muscular endurance.

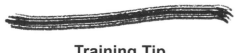

Training Tip

Muscular endurance involves using the muscles continuously over a long period of time. A good supplemental muscular endurance exercise is swimming.

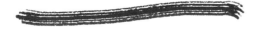

Muscular endurance involves mostly slow-twitch fibers that have the ability to contract over a long period of time. You will realize greater endurance if you approach training when you are fresh and rested. Training under less pleasant circumstances; for example, by eliminating the rest between sets, lifting when your muscles are already fatigued, or dropping down for pushups immediately following an intense run or sprint is also valuable and will call on your muscles to develop endurance.

When you engage in endurance training, your body increases its lactate threshold and preserves carbohydrate stores for extended performance. "Endurance training increases the ability of the muscle to use fat as a fuel and to rely less on carbohydrate energy while it reduces lactic acid and thus increases the lactate threshold. Preserving the carbohydrate stores in the liver and muscle provides the extra glucose needed during the extended performance." (High Performance Sports Conditioning, Bill Foran)

You develop muscular endurance by using lighter weights and more repetitions. A minimum of 12-15 repetitions is recommended with a weight of 40% or less of your 1-repetition maximum, but you might want to go as high as 25 reps per set. You must still use a load that is heavy enough to fatigue the muscles over time. If you can do more than 20-25 repetitions, the weight isn't heavy enough, and you will see little gain. Circuit training, moving from one station to the other, is also a good way to develop muscular endurance. Note that when you go quickly from one exercise to the next, high lactate concentrations in your muscles make it difficult to perform, and you might have to lighten the load in subsequent sets.

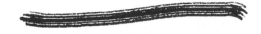

Muscular Endurance Gauge

You can compare your muscular endurance with a person who has greater muscular strength than you. For example, your buddy might be able to bench press twice as much as you, but when you grab a set of light dumbbells and do the same exercise for as many reps as you can without stopping, the person with the greater muscular endurance will prevail, regardless of raw muscular strength.

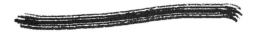

Before starting your muscular endurance training, do a light warm-up of 5-10 minutes to get the blood flowing and ready your muscles for the workout. If running is on today's agenda, start with a walk or slow jog. If weight lifting is on today's agenda, start with some light dynamic stretches, such as arm rotations, trunk rotations, and lunges. You can also warm up with martial arts moves, for example, shadow boxing or forms practice. Try to involve both your lower and upper body.

Right now your main concern is to build a general strength base. Later, when you get into sport specific training, think about what types of muscular endurance your art requires. For example, if it is primarily a kicking art, doing a lot of pushups will not build endurance for kicks. A better way may be to do repeated kicks on a heavy bag or shield.

General Muscular Endurance Exercises

• **Swimming** builds endurance in your whole body and is also a gentle way to start your program. Swim at least 3 times a week. If you are untrained in swimming, start with 8 laps in a 25-meter pool. You do not have to complete the swimming at any particular speed. The idea is to get all the muscles in your body used to working through their entire range of motion. I recommend using the breaststroke, because it gives you great range of motion in both the arms and the legs.

• **Running** builds endurance in your lower body. In addition to squats, I have found running to be one of the better exercises for building lower body strength. Running also strengthens your heart, but you must have the muscular endurance to run for at least 20 minutes in order to gain a noticeable cardiovascular advantage. Start by walking one lap around the track at your local high school (each lap is a quarter of a mile), then jogging one lap, walking one lap, jogging two laps, and walking one lap for cool-down. As you get stronger, increase the walks to a jog and the jogs to a steady run. Shoot for your goal of running one mile; that is, four laps around the track in 12 minutes without stopping or changing your pace.

• **Kicking to failure** builds endurance in your lower body. Choose one of the three basic kicks: front kick, roundhouse kick, or sidekick. Perform the kick in the air as many times as you can without stopping, until you are unable to do another kick with good form. To build static muscular endurance, extend and hold the kick with good form. For example, extend your leg in the front kick position and hold. After 10 seconds, attempt to raise the kick slightly higher and hold for another 10 seconds. You may start by holding on to a wall or table for support.

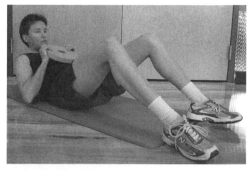

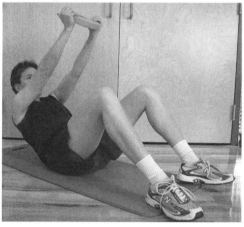

• **Dumbbell punching** builds endurance in your upper body. Start with a set of light handheld weights, 3-5 pounds, and run through a series of punches in the air. For example, punch straight ahead for 20 seconds, straight down for 20 seconds, and straight up for 20 seconds. Repeat 3 times with no stopping or resting. Throw each punch at an even speed and as fast as possible, with full extension in the arm without locking or snapping the elbow. Remember how we talked about that using weighted objects, such as ankle weights or dumbbells, does not improve your kicking and punching skills? The intent of this dumbbell punching exercise is to build upper body muscular endurance, not to improve a specific skill.

A good way to build endurance in the midsection is to bring your torso up a few inches off the floor and hold, then bring it up another inch and hold, then drop back down one inch and hold, never allowing your back to touch the floor. The tension on your abs should be constant for as long as you can muster. To make this exercise more difficult, hold a weight plate to your chest. Also try it with the weight extended away from you at an upward angle.

• **Pushups to failure** build endurance in your upper body. If you are not strong enough to do pushups, you can start against a wall, chair, or other incline. Each pushup should be done with good form to a 90-degree bend at the elbow, and with no sagging in your back or torso. Continue the exercise until you are unable to do another repetition with good form.

• **Situps to failure** build endurance in your midsection. Continue the exercise until you are unable to do another repetition with good form. To build static endurance, hold the situp in the midrange position for as long as you can.

Tips for Improving Muscular Endurance

• Increase dynamic muscular endurance (not necessarily speed) by doing a high number of repetitions against low resistance.

• Simulate the spurts that normally occur within your martial art. For example, go to the track and run or sprint the straightways while walking or jogging the curves. As your endurance improves, make the sprints longer and the jogs shorter.

• Increase endurance by decreasing recovery time. For example, drop down for 10 or 20 pushups immediately following a sprint, and prior to jogging or walking to recover. Or, in the weight lifting gym, do 8 reps on the lat pulldown machine, and then drop down for 8 pushups. Repeat. Maximum recommended recovery time between endurance exercises is 30 seconds.

Muscular strength

Let's talk about the second part of the muscular equation, namely muscular strength. Muscular strength is your ability to generate a high force in a short amount of time, and therefore differs from muscular endurance. But you need to have both. If you only have muscular strength, an opponent with more endurance can outlast you if your first few strikes fail to end the fight. If you only have muscular endurance, you can't deliver a strong blow unless your timing is perfect. Whether muscular strength or muscular endurance is your key priority depends on several factors: Does your art require sudden bursts of energy, as in a 1-strike knockout? Does your art require repeated techniques, as in a 10-minute grappling match?

Your general muscular strength goals involve:

• Preparing your body to accept the greater demands placed upon it when progressing to a martial art specific strength-training program

• Strengthening your muscles, tendons, and ligaments and decreasing the injury risk during your continued strength-training program

Training for muscular strength is an *anaerobic* (without oxygen) activity with the potential for lactic acid build-up in the muscle tissue, which can cause pain. While building your general strength base, start with 2 exercises and 2 sets for each major muscle group, and stretch for a few minutes before and after lifting to help ease pain from lactic acid.

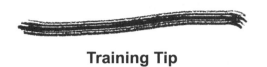

Training Tip

When lifting to develop muscular strength, you need to lift a weight that is heavy enough that you only can do 3-8 repetitions, which is normally around 80% of your 1-repetition maximum. Recommended recovery time for muscular strength training is longer than for muscular endurance training, with 2-3 minutes rest recommended between sets.

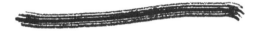

Since muscular strength and muscular endurance are different qualities, if you train strictly for strength, you will not realize much endurance gain, and vice versa. However, there is some carryover where you gain some muscular endurance through muscular strength training. Regardless of what the specific requirements of your art are, your general strength base should include both muscular endurance and muscular strength exercises.

General Muscular Strength Exercises

• **Stair climbing** builds strength in your lower body, and also strengthens your heart. Try it on a stair-climbing machine set steep enough to allow you to bring your thighs parallel with the floor. Or climb real stairs, stepping on every other step.

• **Leg press** builds strength in your lower body. Try it on the leg press machine. Sit down and place your feet on the foot pedal about shoulder-width apart, with your lower and upper leg at a 90-degree angle. Adjust the resistance so that you can do no more than 8 repetitions. Press with your heels (not the balls of your feet) until your legs are extended but not locked at the knees.

• **Lunges** build strength in your lower body. The lunge works each leg separately. Go deep enough to bring your thigh parallel with the floor. Grab a pair of dumbbells for additional weight. Perform each lunge with control and good form.

• **Seated row** builds strength in your upper body. Try it on the rowing machine. Sit down and place your feet against the footrest. Adjust the resistance so that you can do no more than 8 repetitions. Grasp the handles and pull toward you while leaning back slightly.

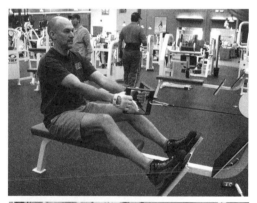

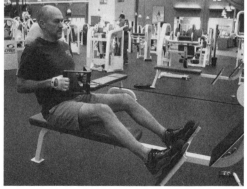

• **Bench press** builds strength in your upper body. Try it on the bench press machine or using a barbell. Lie on the bench and place your feet flat on the floor, and your eyes below the edge of the bar. Adjust the resistance so that you can do no more than 8 repetitions. Grasp the bar slightly wider than shoulder-width, and raise the bar until your arms are extended but not locked at the elbows. If using a barbell, have a friend act as a spotter to help you avoid injury.

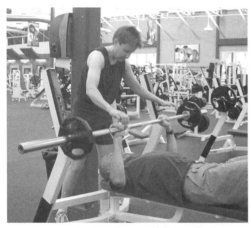

When lifting heavy free weights, use a spotter for safety.

• **Knee-ups** build strength in your midsection. Grasp the bar above your head and hang with your legs straight down. Bring your knees up to your chest. Do not arch your lower back. Use control when lowering your legs. Do not allow gravity to do the job for you. If you can do more than 8 reps with good form, increase the weight by wearing ankle weights, doing the exercise slower, or doing straight-leg raises.

Tips for Improving Muscular Strength

• Do a low number of repetitions against high resistance. If you can do more than 8 reps, increase the load. Work specific muscle groups one at a time.

• Concentrate on controlled movement with good form in both the positive and negative phase of the lift. Do not rely on momentum or gravity to do the work for you.

• As you get stronger, increase the load gradually. Do not increase the reps. Allow 1-2 days of recovery time between training sessions.

Cardiovascular endurance

When you think of cardiovascular endurance, you probably think of how long you can spar without taking a break, or how precisely you can perform a demanding musical form without running out of steam. Cardiovascular endurance is a combination of skill in your sport, aerobic capacity, muscular strength, and genetics.

• **Skill.** A skilled martial artist, with a long background and a lot of experience in his art, knows how to pace himself and relax at the proper moment. He can therefore go longer than a rookie.

• **Aerobic capacity.** This, in combination with muscular strength, allows your muscles to perform for a longer period of time and with greater power output. Muscular strength is tied to endurance performance, since your muscles do the work.

• **Genetics.** You can't do much about your genetic inheritance, so your main focus must be on improving your skill, aerobic capacity, and muscular strength.

Aerobic capacity, or oxygen capacity, differs between individuals, but can be increased through the quantity and intensity of training. Increased aerobic capacity results in increased performance. To increase cardiovascular endurance, push yourself by training at a high intensity level. Any high intensity activity helps you build cardiovascular endurance. I recommend circuit training for your general aerobic base, because it is varied, requires quick switches between exercises, and targets a lot of different muscle groups. Once you have achieved cardiovascular fitness, you can maintain it with less work than it took to achieve it.

Aerobic training should be continuous and preferably involve large muscle groups. Running, swimming, and jumping rope are good choices for the martial arts practitioner. We will look at how strength training affects cardiovascular endurance in greater detail in Chapter 13.

General Cardiovascular Endurance Exercises

• **Running** must be performed at a strong and relaxed pace for at least 20 minutes. Shorter runs of 5 or 10 minutes are not really long enough for building cardiovascular endurance. Make sure you use good foot positioning and a decent stride. Don't allow your feet to drag or "shuffle" across the ground. An appropriate stride makes your running more efficient. Remember, endurance means for the long haul. Make sure you are wearing appropriate running shoes to avoid stress on your feet, ankles, and knees.

• **Swimming** must be performed with effort and intensity. It is often tempting to just lie there in the pool and float around while paddling your hands a little. For the purpose of building cardiovascular endurance, this is not enough. Try alternating strokes; for example, breaststroke for two pool lengths, backstroke for two pool lengths, and sidestroke for two pool lengths. Repeat.

• **Jumping rope** can be done by combining different foot positions, such as alternating feet, jumping forward and backward, and crossing your legs. Do one jump for each swing of the rope, and jump only high enough to allow your feet to clear the rope. There is no need to exaggerate the jump. Avoid large circles with your arms. Keep your shoulders down and your elbows close to your body.

• **Cycling** is a low impact exercise that is gentler on your joints than running or jumping rope. Adjust the seat so that your leg is almost, but not quite, extended at the downward stroke. Grip the handlebars lightly to avoid tension in your neck and shoulders. If on a stationary bike, start with low resistance and increase over time.

• **Kicking the heavy bag** is a good aerobic training exercise. Kick the bag lightly and continuously. For example, start with 1 minute of alternating roundhouse kicks, 1 minute of alternating front kicks, and 1 minute of alternating sidekicks. Then do 2 minutes of combination kicks. Do a "moving rest" by shadow boxing for 2 minutes. Repeat.

• **Continuous forms practice** carries over into your sport specific skills. String together techniques or katas (forms) you have learned, and practice non-stop for 20 minutes. Go through the techniques or forms at different speeds. Start at a medium pace, then at a fast pace, and finally at a slow pace.

Tips for Improving Cardiovascular Endurance

• Work on cardiovascular endurance at least 3 days a week and for at least 20 minutes each time, but feel free to do cardio as often as every day if you have the time and motivation. Watch for overuse injuries, such as sore knees or feet.

• Vary your cardio training with short spurts or sprints. For example, rather than jogging two miles, jog a quarter of a mile, sprint a hundred yards, and jog another quarter of a mile.

• If you do cardio work outside, take your dog along. Soon, your dog will remind you when it is time to do your cardio, and make you feel guilty when you slack.

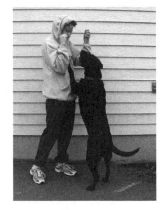

Your dog will get you in shape.

Mobility/flexibility

Flexibility is defined as the range of motion possible around a joint or series of joints. Flexibility differs between people and is influenced by your muscles, ligaments, tendons, and skeletal structure. How flexible you are also depends on how warm your muscles and joints are. It is easier to stretch a joint when it is warm than when it is cold. Warming up prior to stretching increases the blood and oxygen flow to the muscle. "Warming the joint areas produces 20% increase in flexibility, which magnifies the importance of preceding stretching exercises with a warm-up period." (Flexible Perspectives on Stretching, Ken Mannie, www.naturalstrength.com)

There are two types of stretches:

• **Pre-workout stretch**, also called dynamic stretch, which consists of moving type stretches, such as shadow boxing or arm rotations. The pre-workout stretch gets your joints warmed up and ready to move through their entire range of motion. A brief 5-minute warm-up or dynamic stretching routine can get you ready for a harder workout or sparring session. For a short warm-up, I prefer a sport specific routine, such as shadow boxing, which also prepares you mentally for the training.

• **Post-workout stretch**, also called static stretch, which consists of non-moving type stretches, such as toe touches or hurdler stretch. The post-workout stretch is best performed after the workout when the muscles are already warm. I often see martial artists do static stretches at the beginning of their program, when they could achieve more by doing them after the program.

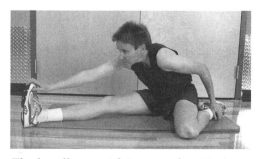

The hurdler stretch is a good static post-workout stretch.

Few would dispute the importance of flexibility. When equating flexibility to the martial arts, we tend to think of leg flexibility. But the benefits that come with flexibility include more than being able to kick to the head. Your arms, shoulders, and trunk also need to be worked through their range of motion if you want the power to perform. We will take a more critical look at flexibility in Chapter 14. For now, let's just establish that it is an important part of your general strength base.

General Mobility/Flexibility Exercises

• **Joint rotations** are dynamic stretches. Stand with your hands hanging at your sides. Flex, extend, and rotate all your joints one at a time. For example, start with your fingers, wrists, elbows, shoulders, neck, trunk, hips, knees, ankles, and toes.

• **Moving lunges** are lower body dynamic stretches that are great for stretching and warming up the hip and hip flexors, glutes, and hamstrings. Step forward in a long stride and into the lunge position, until your lead thigh is parallel with the floor. Bring your rear leg forward and stand back up. Repeat on the other side. Also try the side lunge.

• **Hamstring stretch** is a lower body static stretch. The hamstrings are some of the most injury prone muscles. A good static hamstring stretch is to sit on the floor with one leg straight out. Place the other leg at a 90-degree angle with your foot across the thigh of your straight leg. Reach forward until you feel the stretch. The hamstrings attach to the back of the knee, so you might feel some tightness in this area.

• **Foot, ankle, and quad stretch** is a lower body static stretch. Kneel on the floor with your feet under your body. Lean back and place your hands behind you on the floor. You should feel the stretch in your feet and ankles. If you lean farther back until you are down on your elbows or back, you will also stretch your quadriceps.

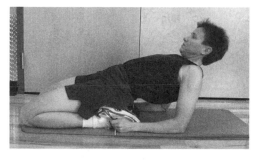

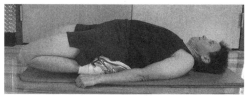

When doing the static quad stretch, use your elbows for support, until you have the flexibility to drop down all the way.

• **Lateral reach** is an upper body dynamic stretch. Stand with your legs about shoulder-width and half apart and your knees slightly bent. Reach as far as you can with one arm laterally across your body. Bring that arm back and repeat on the other side.

• **Shoulder and deltoid stretch** is an upper body static stretch. Reach one arm horizontally across your body. Grab your elbow with your opposite hand and pull your arm across your body. Repeat on the other side.

Tips for Improving Mobility/ Flexibility

• Do dynamic stretches, such as arm and leg rotations, prior to training, and static stretches, such as toe touches or hurdler stretches, after training when the muscles are warm.

• Stretch or move your joints throughout the day, even if just for a few seconds each time. Stretch prior to getting out of bed, after you have been sitting for an hour or longer, and prior to physical work, such as gardening, vacuuming, or cleaning the bathtub.

• Your feet are your foundation and have to carry your weight throughout the day. Rotate your ankles, wiggle your toes, and flex and extend your feet regularly when sitting down.

Rest and recovery

Intense strength training, not just "toning," is recommended for building muscular strength. But intense training involves placing the muscles under considerable stress. In order to allow the muscles to adapt to the higher demands, you must give them adequate time to recover between workouts. Exactly how long you rest between training sessions depends on several factors: the types of exercises you do, your progression, your physical make-up, and your genetics, to name a few, but 48 hours is a good rule of thumb. The muscles need this time to refuel with carbohydrates, which is the main fuel used during an intense workout. Note that you cannot refuel with carbohydrates by eating carbohydrates after having exhausted the muscles. Time is the only viable option. "If the lower body was worked out on Monday, the body's carbohydrate stores were depleted. Even if different muscles are trained on Tuesday, the body hasn't had the necessary 48 hours to fully recover those carbohydrate stores." (A Practical Approach to Strength Training, Matt Brzycki) Resting longer than 3-4 days is not recommended, as the muscles begin to atrophy when not used consistently.

Although your muscles need time to recover from strength training, this is not true regarding cardiovascular training. You can do cardiovascular work every day without negative effects, if you so desire. However, if you do an excessive amount of cardio work, for example, running 10 miles every day, you might have another problem: It might be too hard on your body and cause overuse injuries. Although strength training helps reduce sport related injuries, strength training is in itself an injury risk.

In order to produce strength gains, it is best to train when you are rested. But as a martial artist, there are times when you don't get to choose exactly when you need to use your strength. For example, if you are suddenly attacked on the street, you might need to call on your strength only hours after you have finished a strenuous workout. It is therefore a good idea to experience training under adverse conditions occasionally, when you are tired and near physical exhaustion. At the very least, this will teach you what it feels like to be at the limits of your physical capacity.

When you have finished a training session, you are likely to experience muscle soreness. There are two types of muscle soreness: acute and delayed onset. Acute muscle soreness can be thought of as muscle fatigue and occurs immediately after completion of the exercise. When lactic acid, a metabolic waste product, builds up and can't be removed, you feel pain in the muscles. This type of soreness usually disappears within a couple of minutes of rest. Delayed muscle soreness occurs approximately 24-48 hours after completion of the exercise. This type of muscle soreness is very common, and is normally a response to new demands placed on the body. This is why you need to take it slow in the beginning while your body is getting used to exercise. "If you do want to avoid feeling sore after exercise, the best way is to ease your way into a new training program gradually. After just one bout of exercise, the repair of muscle damage can take up to two weeks." (www.thefactsaboutfitness.com)

Note that feeling muscle soreness is okay and is a normal part of training. However, joint soreness is not normal. If your joints hurt when you are exercising, you need to find out why. You can start by lightening the resistance, using a different exercise, or using a different angle for lifting the weight.

Rest and Recovery Tips

• If you are tired or feel you have over-trained, cut your training time for the next few days, or take a full week off to recuperate. These kinds of breaks are good under the right circumstances, and should not be seen as a lack of discipline.

• Vary your training with maximum effort workouts followed by easier training days. Vary the exercises every few weeks to avoid boredom, burnout, and overuse injuries.

• When recovering between exercises, use an active recovery process that includes gentle stretching, walking around the gym, or moving your arms and legs. Do not sit still on the floor.

Injury rehabilitation

It is almost impossible to escape injury altogether when playing a sport for many years. The most annoying part about being injured, even when the injury is minor, is that you can't practice your art to its fullest while recovering from the injury. Many nagging injuries, such as pulls and strains, heal by themselves with time as long as you give them the chance and avoid aggravating the injury. More serious injuries, such as broken bones or concussions, need a doctor's care. If you sustain an injury, in most cases it is still advisable to continue training in some form or way to prevent muscle atrophy while your injury heals. If you become sedentary or use the fact that you were injured as an excuse not to train, your strength and flexibility will deteriorate.

Whether or not participation in your sport while injured is a good idea depends on the extent and type of injury you have sustained. Each situation must also be evaluated and weighed against the benefits and drawbacks of continued training. For example, finishing a game, competition, or belt promotion despite an injury can give you confidence and command over yourself; you will know that you are not a quitter, and that you can do whatever it takes when called upon. It gives you the proper spirit needed to pursue your art. But be aware that when you train while injured, the rest of your body must make adjustments for the injury, causing you to favor the injured body part. This can place additional stress on the healthy parts of your body and can cause further injury. If you are injured to the point of placing too much stress on your body, you need to take it as a signal to stop until you can participate normally again.

Some injuries require that you take time off from your game for a longer period of time. You may then need additional time to recover your pre-injury conditioning. When your injury has healed, get back into your training slowly, use lower resistance to prevent re-injury, or use shorter training sessions on the injured body part before bringing it back up to your pre-injury strength. Be aware that if you have had a prior injury to a specific body part, you are more likely to suffer a second injury to this same part. For example, I have had two torn hamstrings, one in each leg. It is possible that I have a pre-existing weakness that makes my hamstrings tight, so I need to spend a little extra time on stretching and warming up my hamstrings prior to participating in training that is stressful to this body part.

Injury Tip

If you sustain an injury, it is recommended that you see a sport physician instead of a family practitioner, who understands your needs for physical exercise and strength training and can make recommendations for a viable training and recovery program. A more serious injury might require complete rest.

If you are sick, for example, with a cold, I recommend taking time off from training. Every year, athletes die from inflammation of the heart muscle as a result of engaging in heavy physical training while trying to combat a cold.

If your skill, knowledge, and technical ability outweigh your strength, flexibility, and mobility, you run a greater risk of sustaining an injury. This can happen to athletes who have trained to perfect the mechanics of their art, but who have neglected physical conditioning or strength building. When the demands on your body are greater than what you have prepared for; for example, if you go to competition, sparring, or a belt promotion physically under-prepared, you run a greater risk of sustaining a bruise, sprain, or torn muscle.

The fact that you are engaged in a strength program for your muscles, bones, and tendons decreases the risk of getting a martial arts related injury. But it is still possible that you will sustain an injury due to incorrect lifting technique. Make sure your mind is where it needs to be when you go to the weight lifting gym. If you fail to use correct lifting technique, something as simple as picking up your training log from the floor can result in a back injury. Similar injuries happen every day in the workplace and attest to the fact that it is not how heavy a weight you lift that is the greatest danger, but the lack of correct lifting technique.

You can continue being a weekend martial artist for many years, but if you want to see significant improvement or reach the top, you must take charge of your body and physical conditioning. When you take charge of your training and confront your weaknesses, you have taken the first step toward gaining physical and emotional control of your art and performance. A strong and able body is your foundation for success in the martial arts, regardless of your gender, age, background, or genetic inheritance. Start building your general strength base by going through the suggested strength training circuit.

Circuit training

Circuit training is a great way to build strength, endurance, and flexibility, and involves performing sets of exercises sequentially with only brief rests of 30 seconds between sets. While working to build your general strength base, try the following muscular strength and endurance circuit. The circuit should take 15-20 minutes to complete.

Muscular Strength and Endurance Circuit

Warm-Up Stretches

Joint rotations, 1 minute (see pg. 125)
Moving lunges, 1 minute (see pg. 125)
Lateral reach, 1 minute (see pg. 126)

Strength and Endurance

Leg press, 8 reps (see pg. 88)
Lunges, 20 reps (see pg. 105)
Dumbbell punching, 30 sec non-stop
    (see pg. 119)
Bench press, 8 reps (see pg. 92)
Pushups, 10 reps (see pg. 107)
Seated row, 8 reps (see pg. 95)
Situps, 20 reps (see pg. 110)
Knee-ups, 10 reps (see pg. 122)

Cool-Down Stretches

Foot, ankle, and quad stretch,
    hold for 20-30 seconds (see pg. 125)
Hamstring stretch,
    hold for 20-30 seconds (see pg. 125)
Shoulder and deltoid stretch,
    hold for 20-30 seconds (see pg. 126)

Extra Cardiovascular Edge

1-mile run or 10 minutes
    of continuous forms practice

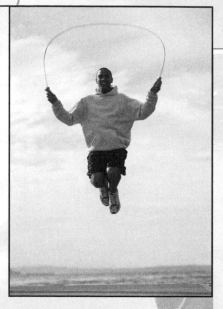

Lower Body Strength

In this section:

- Primary leg functions

- Strong legs = powerful strikes

- The quadriceps

- The hamstrings

- The glutes

- The dorsi flexors (shins)

- The calves

- The feet

Lower Body Strength

In sparring, I have often felt as though my feet were lagging behind my body. When you know you hold the win in your hands, but you can't get your hands to "get there" because your legs won't let you, I'll tell you, it gets real frustrating real fast.

Understand that it is not possible to develop just one part of your body, your hands, for example, and hope for the best. Your great hand speed is useless against a retreating opponent, if your lower body is slow or weak. An under-developed lower body can steal strength from a well-developed upper body, and vice versa. For example, if your legs get tired, your whole body, as far as fighting goes, will get tired. If your arms get tired, your whole body will get tired. Your body is a complete system and should be treated as such. Think of yourself as a whole fighter, not just as somebody with good hands or good legs.

A great deal of power comes through speed, but speed is difficult to attain if you don't have the muscular strength to propel your body forward. Your legs are the driving force and require considerable strength to function, especially when they also have to support the full weight of your body.

Primary leg functions

Strong legs can propel you forward and allow you to place the mass of your body behind your strikes for power. This is one reason good lower body strength gives you stronger upper body techniques. If you lack lower body strength or fail to utilize your legs when punching, you will be an arm-puncher; you will simply throw your strikes quickly (snap the strikes) with no real power behind them. So how quickly you move your foundation is the deciding factor regarding the power of the rest of your body. In other words, hand speed is not that helpful if you are not in position to utilize it. Your legs will get you there.

Primary lower body functions include:

• Supporting the weight of the upper body

• Allowing you to cover distance, for example, when walking or running

• Allowing you to accelerate and increase the power of your upper body, for example, by pivoting

Your legs must be well conditioned since they are used in almost every sport as a means of propulsion. But even if you don't intend to cover any great distances; for example, if you are using only a small ring area for sparring, you must still use your legs to shift position, push off, or move your body in a variety of directions. This applies also to ground arts, such as grappling, that don't use strikes as their primary focus.

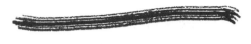

Training Exercise

Get down on the ground on your belly, back, or side and try to shift your weight to different positions without the use of your legs. Try to move short distances of a few inches without the use of your legs. I'm sure you will learn an important lesson: that the legs are absolutely crucial to efficient movement, even on the ground.

Strong legs = powerful strikes

Strength equates to speed, and speed equates to power. Strong legs allow you to set yourself in motion quicker. Strong legs help you throw a strike or kick faster and with less effort. Strong legs are needed for:

• **Trunk twists or pivots**, which originate in your lower body and are used to increase the reach and power of a strike

• **Forward steps**, which allow you to advance on your opponent, close distance, and increase the power of your strikes through momentum

• **Speed**, or how quickly you throw a strike or move your whole body from one position to another

• **Timing**, which is your ability to initiate or throw a strike at a precise moment, which relates to distance and how well you manipulate or adjust that distance

• **Explosiveness**, or the sudden start or stop of motion, which is needed in order to surprise your opponent, overwhelm your opponent, or achieve penetrating rather than pushing power

• **Pushing power**, or the ability to drive with your foundation, which is used when dominating your opponent through body contact

Almost every martial arts move is related to the power of your foundation. This is why they teach us in karate to develop strong stances; this is why they say in boxing, the legs are the first to go; this is why they say, chop down the foundation and the tree will fall. So even if you are concerned mainly with the power of your upper body, it still ties in with the power of your foundation, namely your legs.

Lower body strength is achieved primarily by developing your quadriceps, hamstrings, glutes, dorsi flexors, calves, and feet. The exercises mentioned in this and the next two chapters are suggestions that will give you something to think about. Other exercises are described in detail in Chapters 6 and 7 on weight machines, free weights, and bodyweight exercises.

The quadriceps

The quadriceps muscle group is comprised of four muscles at the front of the thigh, with the primary function of extending and straightening the leg. The legs together with the glutes comprise the biggest muscles of the body, and every sport uses the legs in some way. In martial arts, strong quads are needed for kicking, jumping, running, and throwing. Many of us still tend to neglect lower body workouts while focusing on the upper body. Since the leg muscles are so big, it takes a lot of energy to work the legs; it is strenuous when done right. This may be one reason leg workouts are less popular. Many of us are also more excited about training our upper bodies, often for cosmetic reasons, where we feel a good upper body physique creates a better visual indicator of our strength. While a muscular upper body tempts us to wear tank tops and muscle shirts that allow us to show off the muscles in our shoulders and arms, fewer people naturally look at another person's legs.

Before you start your leg-strengthening workout, it is a good idea to do a few minutes of warm-up to get the blood flowing; for example, five minutes of quick walking on the treadmill, followed by a minute or two of quad stretching, such as grabbing your heel and pulling your foot toward your butt. Try the squat, leg press, and leg extension for strengthening the quadriceps.

• **Squat.** The squat is a multi-joint exercise that also strengthens the hamstrings, and is probably the best exercise for developing the quadriceps. If you have weak knees, you need to exercise caution if squatting to the full position or doing frog hops. (see pg. 103)

The Quad Challenge

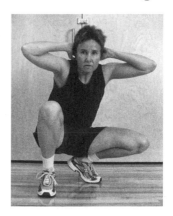

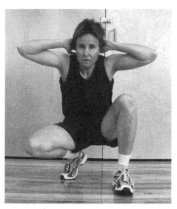

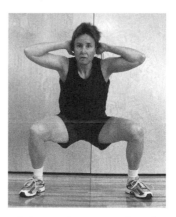

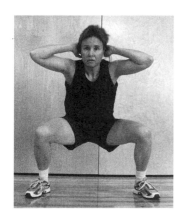

The squat is an excellent exercise for building lower body strength. Squat with your thighs parallel to the floor. Pause for one second at full contraction and repeat.

"Frog hop" from a low squat by alternating your feet forward and back, hands behind your head. Start with 30 total, 15 on each side. Jump up and stand in the squat position with your thighs parallel with the floor for 30 seconds. Repeat two more times. Feel the burn and love it!

- **Leg Press.** This is a safer alternative to the squat, which gives you the option of using a wide range of weights. The leg press is also more stable and therefore slightly less effective than the squat. (see pg. 88)

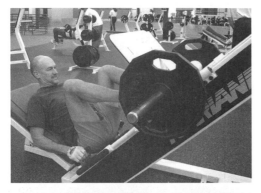

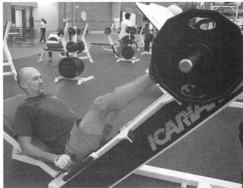

The leg press is a good alternative to the squat.

- **Leg Extension.** This exercise is less effective than the squat and leg press, because it is a single-joint exercise that works the quadriceps in isolation and therefore lacks most sport specific carryover. However, the leg extension is effective for developing the quadriceps specifically for kicks. Another advantage is that the leg extension is gentler on the knee than the squat or leg press. (see pg. 89)

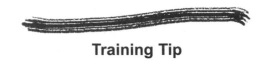

Training Tip

When training the quadriceps, strive to target all four muscles. For example, vary the width between your feet if using the squat or the leg press. A narrow foot placement works the outer thighs more, and a wider foot placement works the inner thighs more.

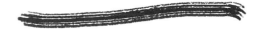

The hamstrings

When thinking about leg strength, many people think only of the quadriceps. As a result, the quads are often over-developed in relation to the hamstrings, which are often neglected. When training the lower body, consider balance between muscle groups and use exercises that specifically strengthen the hamstrings, gluteus maximus (the buttocks, which is the largest muscle in the body and is used, for example, when throwing a sidekick), shins, calves, and feet in addition to strengthening the quadriceps.

The hamstrings are the large muscle group at the back of the thigh. The function of the hamstrings is to bend the knee or extend the hip when moving the thigh to the rear. The hamstrings are used when jumping and running, and less when walking. Some of the most common athletic injuries occur to the hamstrings. I have personally suffered two torn hamstrings, one on each leg, that still give me problems on occasion. The tears happened about a year apart, and both tears occurred near my butt. The first tear was the worst, and made me unable to sit for six months without propping a pillow under my upper leg for support. I was also surprised at how much the injury affected my ability to lift. We think we use mostly the upper body for lifting, but after tearing my hamstrings, my lifting capacity at my job on the ramp at Delta Air Lines was severely hampered for several months.

- **Single Leg Curl.** This is a bodyweight exercise working each leg separately. Get down on all four. Bring one leg off the floor by bending at the knee and bringing your foot toward your head. Keep your leg about shoulder height and your back straight. Do not drop your thigh toward the floor.

The single leg curl does not require access to a gym or equipment. Do 2 sets, 15 reps on each leg in the evening in front of the TV.

- **Machine Hamstring Curl.** This exercise can be done either sitting or lying depending on the type of machine used, and works both legs simultaneously. A drawback is that if one leg is stronger, the weaker leg doesn't get the maximum benefit of the workout. (see pg. 90)

- **Bench Step-Up.** This exercise makes the hamstrings exert force while bearing the weight of your body. Start by standing on top of a bench. Place your bodyweight toward the heel of one foot. Bring your other foot behind your body and off the bench, while bending your supporting leg and lowering yourself toward the floor. Push back up to the starting position by driving with the heel of the foot that is on the bench. Hold dumbbells in your hands for greater difficulty.

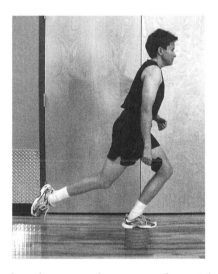

The bench step-up keeps your hamstrings under continuous stress for the duration of the exercise. This also works the quadriceps.

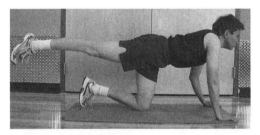

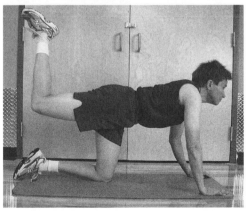

Try the single leg curl, machine hamstring curl, and bench step-up for strengthening the hamstrings.

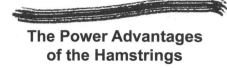

The Power Advantages of the Hamstrings

The origin of the word "hamstring" comes from the Old English "hamm," meaning thigh. "String" refers to the characteristic appearance and feel of the tendons just above the back of the knee. The power advantages of strong hamstrings have been known for a long time. In the past, a sword-wielding knight would disable an opponent by slicing across the back of the thigh. (www.medicinenet.com)

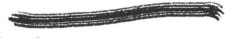

The glutes

Since we spend countless hours sitting on our rear ends, it may seem as though the primary function of the gluteus maximus is to act as a seat cushion. But if you're a martial artist, the primary function of the glutes is hip extension. If you can't extend your hip, you can't throw a sidekick or spinning back kick. The glutes are also used when running, climbing stairs, and jumping rope. Since the legs have less range of motion to the rear than to the front, the glutes generally benefit whenever you work your quadriceps and hamstrings, for example, in the squat or leg press.

If you are not concerned with what others might think, you can work your glutes just about anywhere anytime simply by tightening your butt cheeks and squeezing. Try it while standing in line at the post office or grocery store, or while sitting on the couch in front of the TV. If you're dedicated, you can do hundreds of reps each day. You can also strengthen the glutes through the narrow-stance squat, stability ball lift, and bridge.

• **Narrow-Stance Squat.** This is similar to the regular squat, but in order to target the glutes, keep your feet only about 10-12 inches apart. Squat until your thighs are parallel with the floor. Squeeze your glutes while standing back up. Be aware that as you sit down into the squat, your knees may extend past your toes, which could place stress on the patella tendon. Make sure you are properly warmed up first. You can do this exercise with or without weights.

• **Stability Ball Lift.** This exercise is done lying face down on a bench with your arms wrapped around the bench to hold you in position, and your legs extending straight back off the bench. If you are strong, you can also place your hands behind your head. Grab the stability ball between your feet. Hold the ball about 6 inches off the floor, then raise it an additional 6-12 inches. Your legs should be straight with the muscles in your butt doing the work.

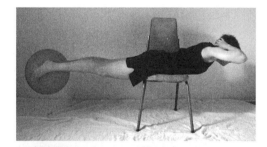

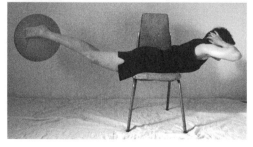

Tighten your glutes and hold the full contraction for a few seconds to avoid using momentum.

• **Bridge.** The bridge can be done with both feet on the floor, or with only one foot on the floor for a greater challenge. When doing the bridge on just one foot, either rest your other foot on your opposite knee or extend your leg into the air. Press your hips up high and squeeze your glutes. Make sure your hips stay level.

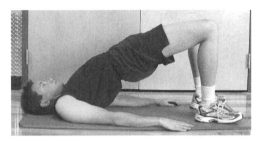

When doing the bridge, press as high as you can so that a straight line is formed between your thigh and your hip. Do not allow your hips to sag toward the floor.

The dorsi flexors (shins)

Have you ever heard of anybody commenting on somebody else's great looking shins? Can you even name one exercise that specifically strengthens the shins? Strengthening the shins is often overlooked at the expense of strengthening the calves. But remember, this is at the risk of causing muscle imbalance and shin splints. Shin splints is a painful overuse injury, usually along the front of the lower leg, and can be caused by running or jumping when your shins are insufficiently prepared to absorb the impact.

Strong shins are especially beneficial in martial arts that involve using the shin as an impact weapon; for example, in Muay Thai, which relies on powerful kicks that impact your opponent's thigh area with your shin. I once knew a man who had an unusually thick muscle running the whole length of his shin. When I asked him about it, he explained that his hobby was hiking, and that the muscle had developed to that degree from flexing the foot toward the shin thousands of times while hiking up steep hills. Try the heel walk, toes over the edge raise, and resistance band tension exercises for strengthening the shins.

• **Heel Walk.** Walk on your heels while flexing your feet toward your shins. Increase the effectiveness of this exercise by walking slowly in small steps and pulling your toes as far back as you can, until they are pointing toward the ceiling. You can do this exercise frequently throughout the day, for example, by walking on your heels whenever you walk around in your home.

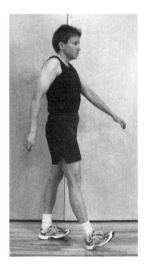

The heel walk is an easy shin-strengthening exercise, without spending extra time at the gym. Stretch your shins for a few seconds between each walk.

• **Toes Over the Edge Raise.** Stand on your heels on a staircase, with your toes extending as far as possible over the edge. Flex your foot and pull your toes toward your shin. Pause for a few seconds at full contraction. Lower your toes. Repeat. You may hold on to the wall or railing to prevent balance loss.

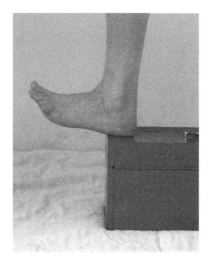

The toes over the edge raise can be done on one foot at a time for increased difficulty.

• **Resistance Band.** Sit on the floor with your legs extended straight out in front of you and wrap an exercise rubber band, or a bicycle tire inner tube, around the top portion of your foot. Attach the other end around the leg of the sofa. Slide back far enough to create tension on the rubber band. Flex your foot toward your shin. Pause for a moment at full contraction. You can also do this exercise sitting on a table with your feet hanging freely, and wrapping a weight over the top of your foot. Now, flex your foot toward your shin.

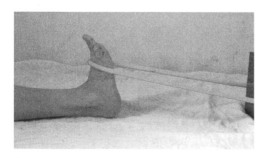

Flexing your foot toward your shin against resistance builds up the dorsi flexors.

The calves

The calves do a lot of work for you every day just by carrying your weight. The calves are comprised of two muscles that together form the Achilles tendon, which assists in flexing the ankle. The calves are involved when walking and running, and specifically when driving the foot forward. Try the toe walk, toe raise, and jump rope for strengthening the calves.

• **Toe Walk.** This exercise is similar to the heel walk shin exercise, except that you walk on your toes instead of your heels (or actually on the balls of you feet). Get as high up as possible on the balls of your feet and walk slowly, taking small steps. Do this exercise frequently throughout the day, for example, when walking around in your home. Stretch for a few seconds between each walk.

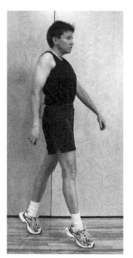

In addition to strengthening the calves, the toe walk is also a good way to practice strength and foot mechanics for the roundhouse kick.

• **Toe Raise.** Stand on a stairway with your heels extending over the edge of the step. Come up on your toes, then lower your heels below the level of the step. Repeat. Pause for a couple of seconds at the high and low ends of the rep. To make this more difficult, work one leg at a time. Try this: Do 10 single leg toe raises on the first step of the stairway, climb up a step and do 10 single leg toe raises on the other foot. Repeat until you have climbed the whole flight of stairs. You may hold on to the wall or railing to prevent balance loss.

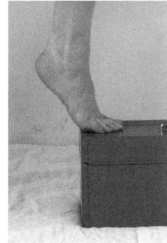

The toe raise, too, can be done on one foot at a time. Hold on to the wall for balance.

• **Jump Rope.** This is an intense aerobic exercise that also strengthens the legs, specifically the calves and the hamstrings. Start by jumping on both feet together. Then vary by jumping on one foot at a time. Jumping rope is a bit more time consuming than the other calf exercises, but can be done in lieu of running to knock off part of your cardio workout simultaneously.

The feet

When going through athletic literature, I hardly ever read or hear about the necessity to strengthen the foot, which surprises me since the foot is one of the most important and complex parts of the human body. The foot allows you to walk, run, shuffle, and kick. Without the foot, you would be pretty limited in your skills, at least the way most martial artists train.

The foot is capable of eight different moves: dorsal flexion, plantar flexion, adduction, abduction, inversion, eversion, toe flexion, and toe extension.

Dorsal flexion = top part of the foot brought toward the shin

Plantar flexion = top part of the foot extended (stretched)

Adduction = feet (toes) turned to the inside

Abduction = feet (toes) turned to the outside

Inversion = sole of the foot tilted to the inside (top part to the outside)

Eversion = sole of the foot tilted to the outside (top part to the inside)

Toe flexion = toes curled under

Toe extension = toes extended and curled upward

You can easily exercise all eight moves of the foot while sitting in front of the TV.

Hint: When walking or running, be aware of your foot placement. Many people tend to run with their toes pointed slightly to the outside, placing undue stress on the inside edges of the feet. The stress of running should be along the center of the foot and through the big toe, not toward the inside of the big toe or toward the little toes.

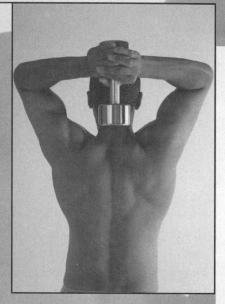

Upper Body Strength

In this section:

- Why you need a strong upper body

- Avoiding muscle imbalance

- The upper back

- The lower back

- The shoulders

- The biceps

- The triceps

- The forearms

- The hands

- The neck

Upper Body Strength

Training Exercise: Go to the weight lifting gym and observe the types of exercises the clientele are doing. Don't worry, you don't have to do any yourself, at least not right now. Just bring a fruit juice or sports candy bar and sit back and observe.

First, look at the gender mix. Approximately what percentage is male vs. female? If there is an uneven mix, why do you think this is? There might not be a definite answer, and the reason I ask is to stimulate thought and help you determine your reasons for lifting weights as opposed to going to aerobic class. In general, I have found the following:

• More men than women lift weights, and more women than men go to aerobic class or use aerobic machines, such as elliptical trainers, rather than lifting weights.

• Men work their upper bodies more than their lower bodies, and women work their lower bodies more than their upper bodies.

• Both men and women do more pushing type exercises than pulling type exercises; for example, the bench press (pushing exercise) vs. the pull-up or row (pulling exercise).

• Both men and women tend to favor lying on their backs a lot when lifting weights, for example, bench press vs. pushup.

Upper body strength is achieved primarily by developing your upper back, lower back, shoulders, biceps, triceps, forearms, hands, and neck.

Why you need a strong upper body

A strong upper body benefits you because it makes you look powerful, which gives you a psychological advantage. In more practical terms, you need upper body strength to attack and defend effectively. In the martial arts, upper body strength is needed for:

• **Striking.** Although finger whips and other strikes to sensitive targets may not require a lot of strength, a good old-fashioned punch is still one of the most popular strikes. A wimpy strike makes your opponent lose respect for you. This is true whether you are in the training hall or on the street.

• **Defense.** A strong upper body helps you keep your ground and block your opponent's offense at a decreased risk of injury to yourself. When you strength-train, it is not only your muscles that become stronger, but also your bones. You can therefore absorb the power of your opponent's offense better.

• **Gripping and Twisting.** Many martial arts employ gripping or grappling techniques ranging from a simple arm or wrist grab to a full grappling match. Hand and forearm strength are important in order to secure a good grip. Arm and shoulder strength allow you to execute more forceful twists of your opponent's arm, leg, or joint, especially if you are up against a person with bigger limbs than you.

• **Holding and Pinning.** Good upper body strength allows you to use momentum to move your opponent back, pin him to a wall or floor, or hold him down.

Technique vs. Strength Debate

Arm strength alone is not the primary tool used when striking, holding, or pinning. For example, correct body mechanics and use of weight and momentum play a crucial role. But a stronger opponent can easily defeat your wimpy upper body, even if you use correct mechanics. Rarely do we see a muscularly weak person defeating a bigger adversary. There are no secrets to the martial arts and, just as in any other sport, strength benefits you sometimes more than good technique.

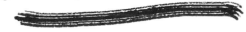

Avoiding muscle imbalance

As you continue your observations at the gym, you may find that many people work only one side of their body. No, I'm not talking about the left side vs. the right side. I'm talking about the chest but not the back, the arms but not the legs, the biceps but not the triceps, or pushing but not pulling. You will find that this muscle imbalance usually favors the chest and the biceps over the back and the triceps, and that it usually favors pushing type moves over pulling type moves. Very seldom do you observe the reverse type of imbalance. In addition, most of us completely ignore the neck.

To avoid muscle imbalance, include exercises that work both the front and the back of your upper body, and do a variety of exercises including pushing and pulling routines. For example, do pull-ups for vertical pulls, and rows for horizontal and diagonal pulls; do overhead presses for vertical pushes, and pushups and bench presses for horizontal pushes. Note that the pull-up is too difficult for starters. In fact, it takes the average man or woman one full year of training to be able to do even one full straight-arm palms forward pull-up. I still recommend that you train in the pull-up because, if you master it, it will give you great confidence in your upper body strength capacity.

Some training manuals suggest that if you lack the strength to do a pull-up, do pulldowns instead. I disagree. Although the pulldown appears to utilize identical motion, it has one major flaw: It does not prepare you for controlling and manipulating your own bodyweight. It is therefore less sport specific than the pull-up, which requires you to lift your own weight in an unstable situation; for example, if you need to climb a rope or a high fence to get away from an adversary. If you are unable to do a pull-up, it is better to train in assisted or negative pull-ups than in pulldowns.

Upper Body Strength Suggestion

Most martial arts rate high in need for upper body strength and muscular endurance. Upper body strength does not only relate to throwing punches or wrestling your opponent to the ground. Your first goal should be to manipulate and move your own body effectively. A challenging and useful goal you can set for yourself is to train until you can lift up and hold your own bodyweight; that is, until you can do at least one full pull-up and hold the up position for at least three seconds.

The upper back

Since the trapezius and latissimus dorsi are the most prominent muscles of the upper back and are used in all lifting and pulling moves, it is crucial to train the upper back at least as much as you train the chest. Try the row, pulldown, and chin-up for strengthening the upper back.

• **Upright Row.** Grab a barbell in an overhand grip (palms of your hands turned toward you). Your grip should be slightly narrower than shoulder-width. Lift the bar straight up to your chin while allowing your wrists to flex and your elbows to point to your sides. Keep your elbows above the bar. Squeeze your shoulder blades together at the top of the lift. Keep the bar close to your body and do not jerk the bar up.

• **Pulldown.** Sit on a bench and grab the pulldown bar in a wide grip. Pull the bar down toward your chest. You might need to lean back slightly in order to keep the bar close to your body. Make sure your arms are extended fully when you return the bar to the original position.

• **Chin-Up.** The chin-up is a bodyweight exercise; in other words, it does not rely on external weights for resistance. Grab the chin-up bar with the palms of your hands facing toward you (if you do pull-ups, you grab the bar with the palms of your hands facing away from you. Most people find the pull-up tougher than the chin-up). Start in the straight-arm position and pull yourself up until your chin is above the bar. Lower yourself all the way down to the straight-arm position. Do not lock your elbows. If you cannot do chin-ups, try negatives and, if possible, hold your weight for a few seconds at the halfway point.

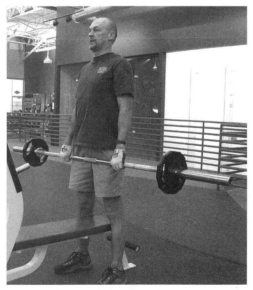

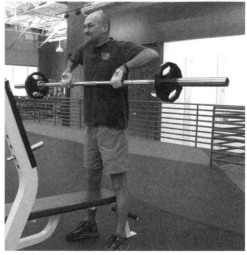

The lower back

Lower back strength training is another area that is often neglected. The muscles in the lower back are crucial to maintaining good posture, and include parts of the latissimus dorsi, the spinal erectors, and parts of the glutes. A strong lower back is required when lifting or picking up an object from the ground. Try the back extension, good morning, and deadlift.

• **Good Morning.** Stand with your legs straight and about shoulder-width apart. Place a staff (a bo-staff, for example) across your shoulders. Bend at the waist until your trunk is parallel with the floor. The movement should be in your hips with your back straight. Come back to the upright position. Keep your legs straight but not locked, your head up, and your shoulders back throughout the exercise. As you master the movement, you can increase the weight by using a barbell instead of a bo-staff.

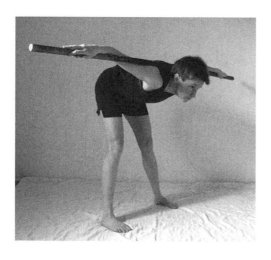

The good morning is a great lower back exercise. Be very careful and make sure you master the movement before increasing the weight.

• **Back Extension.** Lie on the floor or on a bench with your upper body extending over the edge of the bench. Place your hands behind your head and raise your upper body until your chest is off the floor, or until your back is arched.

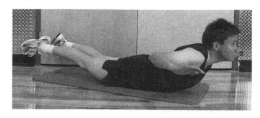

When doing back extensions on the floor, pretend that you are swimming in the ocean and bobbing on a huge wave.

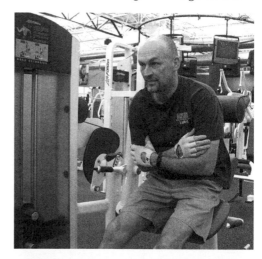

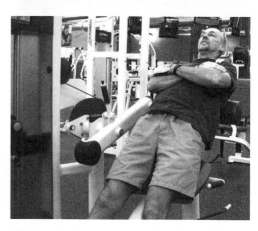

Also try back extensions against resistance on a machine.

• **Stiff-Legged Deadlift.** The deadlift

involves the lifting of a weighted barbell off the floor. Stand with your feet about shoulder-width apart and bend forward at the hips. Keep your back straight and your legs slightly bent. Grab the barbell with your hands in alternate grips (one hand palm forward, the other palm backward). Lift the bar by straightening your hips. Keep your back straight and the bar close to your shins throughout the lift. At the end of the lift, the barbell should be about level with your hips. This exercise also targets your glutes and hamstrings.

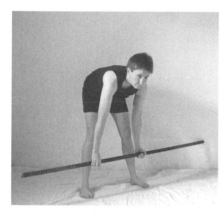

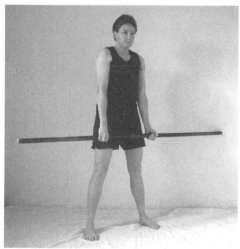

The stiff-legged deadlift, too, can be done with a lightweight staff before increasing the weight.

The shoulders

The shoulders are capable of rotating the arm in several planes. The martial arts, especially the striking arts, require repetitive movements of the shoulders and, therefore, good shoulder strength. Strong shoulders also protect against dislocation injuries that can easily happen in the grappling arts. In order to function properly, all muscles of the shoulders must be strengthened. Try the military press, lateral raise, and shoulder rotation.

• **Military Press.** You can do the military press with a barbell, dumbbells, or weight machine. Position the weight even with your shoulders and grab the bar with the palms of your hands facing forward. Press straight up above your head until your arms are straight. Lower the weight and repeat.

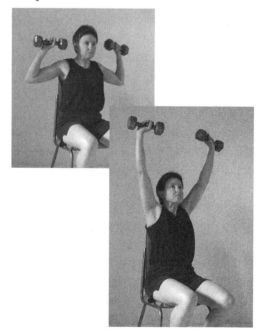

Most people find the military press tougher than the bench press, because the weight is pressed straight up, not at an angle.

• **Lateral Raise.** Stand with your feet about shoulder-width apart. Hold a dumbbell in each hand. The palms of your hands are facing in toward your body, so that the short ends of the dumbbells are facing to the front and back. Raise the weights straight up and to your sides, until your arms are extended straight out from your shoulders.

• **Shoulder Rotation.** This exercise prepares you for throwing a strong back fist. Use a cable machine, resistance band, or dumbbells if you are lying on the floor. To use the cable machine, stand sideways, bring the hand that is farthest away from the cable in front of your body and grab the handle. Bend your arm at the elbow to form a 90-degree angle. Keep your upper arm close to your body, rotating your forearm to the outside. You can also do this exercise rotating your forearm to the inside by grabbing with the hand closest to the cable.

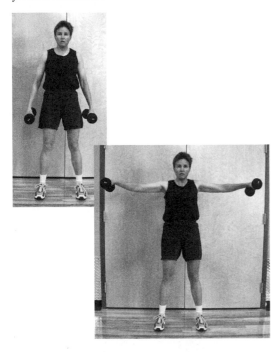

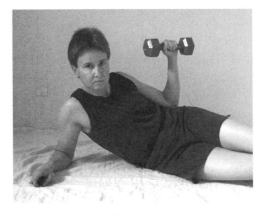

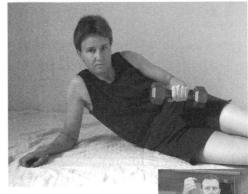

Do not shrug your shoulders on the lateral raise; keep them down throughout the lift.

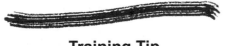

Training Tip

Once you know which particular muscle group is involved the most in a movement, such as a pushup or a pull-up, you will seem stronger if you can focus on working and tightening this particular muscle group. When doing pull-ups, rather than pulling with your arms only, squeeze your upper back muscles together.

Shoulder rotations with resistance increase the type of strength needed for throwing a strong back fist. Use dumbbells for variation.

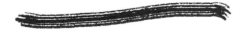

The biceps

The biceps are involved when bending the arm. The biceps are one of the more popular muscle groups to develop. After all, who doesn't want a set of "big guns?" The biceps curl is the typical biceps exercise, and you can do several variations to target different parts of your biceps while avoiding boredom. When doing the biceps curl, keep your elbows close to your body and avoid using momentum or "throwing your upper body to the rear." Do not lift with your shoulders. To reach full biceps potential, twist your wrist inward throughout the movement of the curl. Try the incline bench barbell curl, dumbbell curl, and resistance band exercise.

• **Incline Bench Barbell Curl.** Grab a barbell and place your arms over the edge of an incline bench. The bench should extend past your elbows and support your triceps. Bend your arms and raise the barbell toward your shoulders, but do not lift with your shoulders. The greater the incline on the bench is, the more difficult the exercise.

• **Dumbbell Curl.** Grab a dumbbell in each hand and do biceps curls by bending your arms and raising the weights toward your shoulders. Pause for a second at full contraction. You can vary the routine by using a two-count on the positive phase and a four-count on the negative phase, or vice versa.

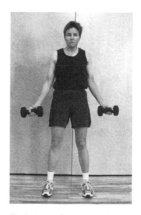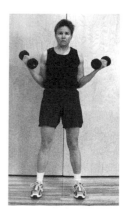

Raising the weights at an angle to the side, while keeping your elbows close to your body, targets a different part of the muscle.

• **Resistance Band.** Stand on the resistance band and grab one end in each hand. Bend your arms and bring the handles up toward your shoulders by bending your arms at the elbows. Start with the palms of your hands facing toward you. As you bring the handles up, rotate your hands 180 degrees so that they are still facing toward you at full contraction.

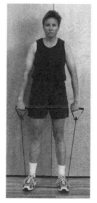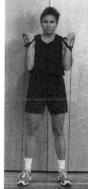

The resistance band is a great alternative when you are traveling.

The triceps

The triceps are involved in the extension of the arm and are needed, for example, when throwing a punch. You know that you have neglected training the triceps when you have flabby bags of skin hanging from your upper arms. Try the triceps extension, chair dip, and triceps pushup.

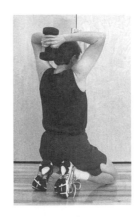
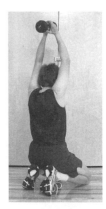

The French press is a good alternative. Hold a dumbbell with both hands behind your head. Bend your arms to 90 degrees. Raise the weight straight up until your arms are fully extended.

• **Triceps Extension.** Grab a dumbbell and stand slightly hunched over with your free hand on your knee, or with your knee on a bench. Bring the weight up until your arm is bent 90 degrees at the elbow. Extend your arm straight back. Do not drop your shoulder or allow your arm to swing. Repeat.

• **Chair Dip.** Place your hands on a chair behind you, with your butt hanging over the edge of the chair. Keep your legs extended and your feet on the floor. Bend your arms and lower your butt toward the floor. Press back up. To make this exercise more difficult, use parallel bars and keep your feet completely off the floor.

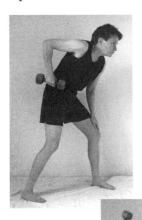

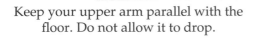

Keep your upper arm parallel with the floor. Do not allow it to drop.

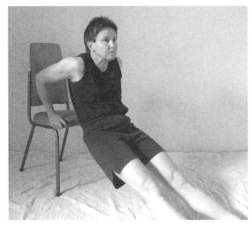

Bend your arms to 90 degrees for maximum effort.

• **Triceps Pushup.** Get down in the pushup position with your hands forming a triangle under your chest. Lower yourself toward the floor until your chest is touching your hands (if you can, this is tough). Press back up and repeat. To make this exercise easier, place your hands on a bench or chair instead of on the floor. To make it more difficult, place your feet on a chair.

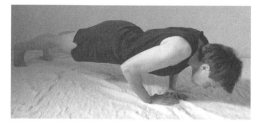

Keep your back straight. Don't allow your body to sag.

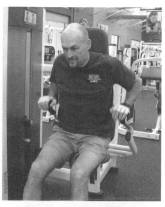

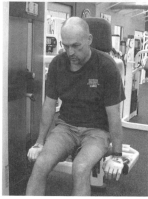

The triceps pushdown machine is a good alternative, if you are at the gym.

The forearms

Most movement that involves any use of your hands also works your forearms. This includes twisting or bending your wrists, and grabbing or gripping. I have found that my job on the ramp at Delta Air Lines is great for developing strong forearms. I grab and lift around a thousand bags every day, and I have been doing this job for twenty years. In the martial arts, you need strong forearms for grappling, gripping, locking, and blocking. Strong forearms give you a stronger grip, and are less prone to injury when blocking an opponent's punch or kick. If somebody with strong forearms grabs you, you will know what I mean. Try the wrist curl, wrist rotation, and nunchakus.

• **Wrist Curl.** Lay your forearm on a table with your hand and wrist extending over the edge, palm up. Grab a light dumbbell, 5-10 pounds, in your hand. Curl your wrist upward. Repeat. Next, rotate your arm over so that your palm is facing down. Curl your wrist upward.

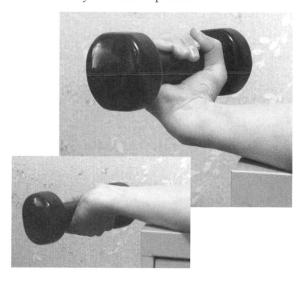

The wrist curl is a simple and effective forearm exercise you can do, for example, while talking on the phone.

• **Wrist Rotation.** Bend your arm 90 degrees, palm facing up, and hold a light dumbbell, 3-5 pounds, in your hand. Rotate your forearm inward until your palm faces down. Rotate your forearm back outward to the starting position. Repeat.

• **Nunchakus.** Work a set of nunchakus for 5-10 minutes. The heavier the nunchakus are and the tighter the movement, the greater the forearm workout. Swing and twirl the nunchakus in both directions.

The hands

Gripping strength is often overlooked. But if you think about it, you need quite a bit of gripping strength in the martial arts. You use it when grabbing and throwing, when pulling and pushing, when twisting and pinching, when applying a joint lock, and when wielding a weapon at high speed. In addition, your ability to grip and maintain your grip communicates a psychological advantage that prevents your opponent from escaping.

Your gripping fingers are your smaller fingers, namely the little finger and ring finger. Your gripping strength is along this line of your hand. This is in contrast to your thumb and index finger, which are used for fine motor skills, such as pointing or manipulating a pencil.

Not all gripping is done the same way. For example, crushing and pinching require different kinds of gripping strength. When you crush, you use mainly the palm of your hand as a base, with your little finger and ring finger pulling in toward your hand. When you pinch, you use mainly your fingertips and thumb. Both types of grips are useful in the martial arts.

There are a number of gripping exercises that also develop your forearms. Try the newspaper ball, towel twist, and crushing grip strengthener.

• **Newspaper Ball.** Place one full sheet of newspaper on the floor. Place your hand in the center of the paper, spread your fingers, and start wadding up the paper into your hand. Don't stop until you have formed a newspaper ball in your hand, and your hand completely envelopes the ball. This is tougher than you think. Try it!

• **Towel Twist.** Grab a bath towel in each end and start twisting in opposite directions, until the towel is twisted completely tight. This gives your wrists a great workout. You can also do this exercise by wringing out a wet towel.

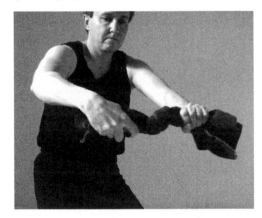

• **Crushing Grip Strengthener.** This is the spring loaded grip strengthener you can buy for a few bucks at a sporting goods store. Keep it in your car and work alternating hands each time you get to a stoplight.

There are several simple grip-strengthening devices on the market; for example, the crushing grip strengthener, a piece of foam designed for gripping, or a ball of clay or putty.

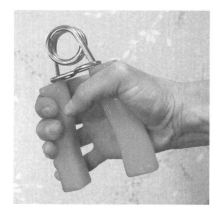

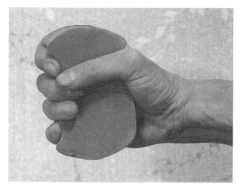

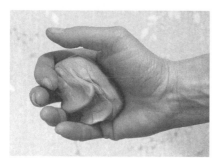

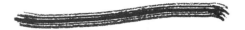

Pinch Grip Training Tip

Get a teardrop shaped object of some weight; a plumb bob, for example. Grip the pointed end between the tip of your thumb and fingers and lift up. When you can do this with your thumb and all four fingers, try it with only your thumb and three, two, or one finger.

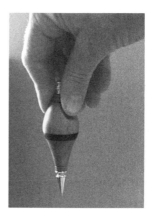

Gripping the tapered end of a plumb bob between your thumb and fingers helps you build pinching grip strength.

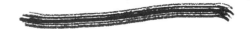

Remember how we have talked about working opposing muscle pairs? If you have good gripping strength; that is, the kind of strength that allows you to close your hand, wouldn't it also be appropriate to have the kind of strength that allows you to open your hand? For example, if somebody grabs your hand and squeezes, can you counter his move and free yourself simply by opening your hand? To train this type of strength, make a fist and place it in the palm of your other hand. Try to open your fist against the resistance of your other hand. This is an exercise that you can easily work while sitting in front of the TV.

The neck

The neck is often neglected in strength training, despite the fact that a strong neck is crucial to martial artists taking strikes to their heads, or to grapplers experiencing intense strain on their necks. The neck moves in six directions: upward tilt, downward tilt, left tilt, right tilt, left turn, and right turn. All of these directions can be combined through circular rotation of your head. The neck is targeted in:

• **Contact Competition Matches that Allow Strikes and Kicks to the Head.** Blows to the head in full contact arts can cause whiplash injuries or knockouts that a strong neck helps protect against.

• **Neck Cranks and Neck Takedowns.** Many takedowns use neck cranks to get the opponent on the ground. Neck cranks present a risk of injury that a strong neck helps protect against.

• **Grappling and Chokes.** If you are choked, a strong neck or tightening of the neck muscles can buy you significant time or allow you to defeat your adversary.

• **Street Fights Involving Strikes to the Throat.** Even a direct strike to your windpipe can be withstood better if you have strong neck muscles you can tighten at the right time.

Training Tip

A neck injury could be debilitating for life. When strengthening the neck, keep in mind that it is a sensitive part of your anatomy, so you want to start out with very little resistance, generally just the weight of your head, and use controlled movement with no snapping or jerking. Do at least two neck exercises along with your upper body training.

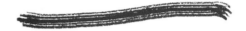

You use your arms and legs continuously throughout the day, so normal range of motion in your limbs usually don't create soreness. The same is not true when it comes to the neck. Although you probably turn your head side-to-side a number of times throughout the day, you are less likely to do head tilts forward, back, or to the sides. When you have completed your first neck-strengthening workout, you will probably feel considerable muscle soreness the next day. I am generally not supportive of neck strengthening exercises using a rubber band or pulley, because I feel the risk of inadvertently applying a snapping move to the neck is too great. The decision is yours, but I recommend neck exercises that are more carefully controlled. Try the weighted neck flexion, weighted lateral flexion, and neck nod and head roll.

• **Weighted Neck Flexion.** Lie on your back on a bench or stability ball with your head extending over the edge of the bench. Grab a weight plate, 5 or 10 pounds for example, and place it on your forehead while holding on to the weight with both hands. You can place a towel between your forehead and the plate to make this more comfortable. Bring your head up until your chin touches your chest. Return your head back down below the horizontal position and repeat.

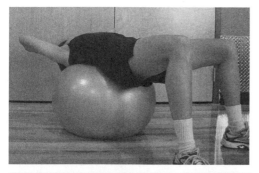

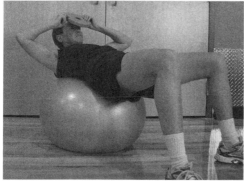

Weighted neck flexion is a controlled neck strengthening exercise. If the weight becomes too heavy, you can easily lift it off your forehead.

• **Neck Nod and Head Roll.** Lie on your back on the floor, bringing your chin toward your chest in a nod. Drop your head back down. Repeat. Do a set of 10 at a pace of about one per second. Next, do a four-count: Bring your chin toward your chest, bring your left ear toward your left shoulder without dropping your head back down, drop your head down to the center, bring your head up with your right ear toward your right shoulder, bring your chin toward your chest. Repeat 10 times in each direction.

• **Weighted Lateral Flexion.** Lie on your side on a bench or stability ball with your head extending over the edge of the bench. Grab a weight plate, 5 or 10 pounds for example, and place it on the side of your head while holding on to the weight with one hand. Tilt your head with your ear toward your shoulder. Return your head back down below the horizontal position and repeat. Do this exercise on both sides.

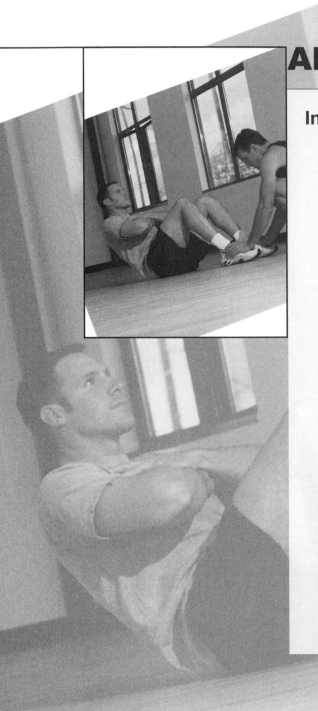

Abdominal Strength

In this section:

- Why you need strong abs

- Abdominal strength when striking

- How often should you work the abs?

- Training the abs

- The lower abs

- The obliques

- The upper abs

Abdominal Strength

What we generally refer to as the trunk, core, midsection, or abdominals is not an isolated muscle group, but is the connective link or medium for transferring movement and power from the lower body to the upper body, or from the legs to the arms. Abdominal strength is needed for almost every athletic movement, so this muscle group must not be ignored while training your lower and upper body separately. Abdominal strength is critical in sports that involve striking, throwing, and twisting; in other words, the martial arts.

The abs (rectus abdominis) is one big muscle, but we normally think of it as several sections divided into the lower abs, upper abs, and obliques extending along the sides of your body. Although ab exercises stress the whole muscle to some degree, when choosing your ab routine, it is recommended that you start with exercises that target the stronger part of the muscle, working toward the weaker part. This gives each part of the abs the maximum benefit of the workout.

Normally, you would work your lower abs, obliques, and upper abs in that order. If you reverse the order and start with the upper abs, fatigue in this part of the muscle may result in inability to work the lower abs to their full potential. In general, exercises that involve movement of your legs target the lower portion of the abs, and exercises that involve movement of your upper torso target the upper portion of the abs.

Train your abs with enough intensity to cause muscle soreness. In other words, it is not the number of crunches or how often or long you do each exercise that is important, but how much resistance you use.

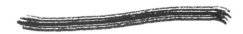

Six-Pack

Washboard abs, although impressive, have more to do with a lean body than with strength, and the only way you can get your abs to show is by reducing the fat around your midsection considerably. While a lean midsection benefits you from a psychological standpoint, since a fit look is intimidating to your opponent, strong abs, even if they don't show, give you sport specific benefits.

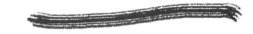

Why you need strong abs

Next time you go to the gym, pay attention to what others are working on, and you will most likely find that it is not the abs. Since the midsection is involved in some way in just about every move you make, developing the abs should be one of your primary concerns. A strong midsection gives you speed and power, and helps stabilize the body. The abs are involved in:

• **Striking and Kicking.** Strong abs allow you to transfer strength from your feet and legs to your arms and hands, giving you the ability to power up and accelerate your strikes.

• **Twisting.** Strong abs allow you to execute quick twists; for example, when throwing an opponent over your hip, or when wielding a weapon such as a stick, staff, sword, or nunchaku. The force transfers from your lower body through your midsection to your arms and into the weapon, resulting in the acceleration of the weapon. This is called the *kinetic-link principle*.

• **Takedowns and Throws.** Strong abs allow you to throw weighted objects with force, for example, an opponent or a weapon, such as a rock or a knife.

• **Grappling.** Strong abs allow you to fight more effectively from the ground, for example, when bridging and unbalancing an opponent who is straddling you.

We often tend to work the abs at the end of the training session; that is, if we have any time and energy left over. If you find that you are missing ab work most of the time, you may want to start with the abs rather than saving them until the end.

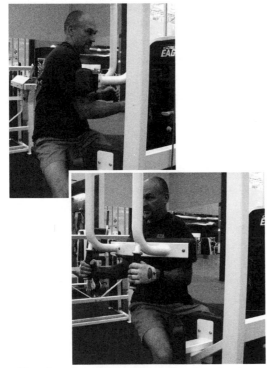

Try the ab twist machine for developing powerful trunk twists.

Abdominal strength when striking

Most martial arts use strikes in some form or way. A strong strike relies on bodyweight, momentum, pivot, and explosiveness. We know that leg strength and upper body strength play a crucial role regarding power, and most of us learn that pivoting should be used in the correct execution of a punch. Your trunk must therefore be strong to allow you to execute a forceful pivot.

Some conditioning coaches have you do crunches at a fast speed to teach you to contract your abs suddenly. Others throw a medicine ball at your abdomen to get you to tighten your abs at the right time and absorb the power of a blow. When training the abs for forceful pivots, I recommend throwing the medicine ball to your partner or against a brick wall, instead of taking the force on your abs. Tighten your abs every time you throw or pass the ball to your partner, and pay attention to the additional power you acquire.

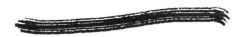

Training Tip

When pivoting to throw a strike or weighted object, you achieve more explosiveness and power if you also contract your abs simultaneously.

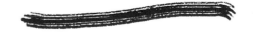

How often should you work the abs?

How often you train the abs is a widely debated issue. Some say to train the midsection every day, and others say that once a week is the best. Still, others say to train to failure and then not train again until the soreness is gone. Others say that any exercise that involves the ab muscles (which are most movements to some degree) gives the abs enough training, and that it is unnecessary to do additional ab work. Still, others say abs are made in the kitchen, and you can get good abs only by dieting and not by training. "If your goal is to develop your abs either for bodybuilding or sport performance, then you should only train them 2-3 days per week using more advanced techniques, e.g. weighted incline crunches performing 6-8 sets." (Robert DiMaggio, www.ironmagazine.com)

Whether you train the abs at the beginning or end of your workout is also a debated issue. If you train the abs at the end of the workout, you risk overlooking good core training because you are already tired from working your lower and upper body. However, if you train the abs at the beginning of the workout, you might fatigue them to the point that it interferes with other exercises, such as squats or pushups. When I go to the gym, I usually train the abs at the end of the workout; when I go to karate class, I usually train the abs at the beginning of the workout.

Training the abs

I have found the abs to be one of the more challenging muscle groups to train because if you don't diet and cut the fat, it won't show externally that you have strong abs. Although a six-pack that shows is not crucial to strength (since one that doesn't show could be just as strong), it serves as a motivational factor, making you want to work the abs harder when you see progress. I also have a hard time finding a good ab exercise that is both time economical and gives me a good burn. Hanging straight-leg raises is such an exercise, but is not convenient to do if you don't have a bar to hang from. Follow these training suggestions when working the abs:

• When training the midsection, think of it as training the entire trunk, including the back and sides of your body.

• Do ab work with controlled speed in both the positive and the negative phase. If you use explosive moves you create momentum and the exercise becomes less efficient, because the muscles don't need to tense throughout the entire range of motion.

• When doing situps, crunches, or leg lifts, focus on drawing in your abs rather than pushing them out. This helps you press your lower back into the floor, keeping it from arching, and eventually allowing you to do these exercises without the support of your hands under your lower back. Place a 10-pound weight plate on your abs to remind you to draw them in.

• Don't do situps or leg lifts with straight legs until you have built up a very good strength base. Some people say that you should never do straight leg situps. My opinion is that such advice is a bit extreme, but I recommend proceeding with caution. Straight leg situps do increase the risk of injury since they might cause you to arch your back if you lack significant strength. Either bend your legs or place your hands under your lower back.

• Don't allow your abs to rest during a set of exercises. For example, if doing situps or crunches, don't allow your shoulders to touch the floor between each rep. You want to keep constant tension on your abs throughout the set. If doing hanging leg or knee raises, don't straighten your legs completely on the downward motion. This would relieve the stress on your abs and make the exercise easier.

• Do situps without a partner holding your feet. If your partner holds your feet, or if you hook your feet under a bar or sofa, you can cheat by using your legs to pull yourself up. You know when this happens because your legs, and not your abs, are getting tired.

A question that is often raised is whether the full situp is good for building abdominal strength, or if it is better to do a partial situp. The abs are used primarily during the first 30 degrees of the situp. Then the hip flexors take over, which are strong muscles with the function of bringing the legs toward the upper body, or the upper body toward the legs. So full situps don't work the abs more than partial situps. However, there is no harm in doing them. Note that the rectus abdominis muscle also works through about 15 degrees of spinal extension, which means that in order to get full benefit from your ab workout, you should avoid lying on a hard floor that prevents you from extending your spine. This is one reason the stability ball is a good ab training device.

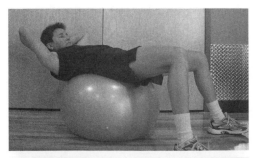

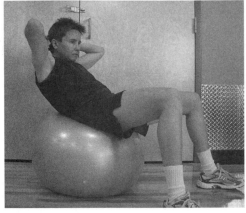

The stability ball allows you to work your abs through 15 degrees of spinal extension. Since you are training on an unstable surface, it forces you to tense your muscles harder in order to control the movement. Greater tensing translates into a greater strength advantage and greater sport specific strength.

The lower abs

Since the abdominals is one muscle group, it is not possible to contract just one part of the muscle independently. However, we often divide the muscle into the lower abs, upper abs, and obliques so that we can focus our exercises without tiring one part of the muscle prematurely. It is recommended that you do lower ab exercises first, followed by oblique exercises, followed by upper ab exercises. The lower abs are challenged more when you do ab work that involves the lower body; for example, the reverse crunch. The obliques are challenged more when you do ab work that involves twisting; for example trunk rotations or diagonal crunches. The upper abs are challenged more when you do ab work that involves the upper body; for example, situps.

When doing lower ab exercises, lift your head and shoulders off the floor. This makes the exercise more difficult and decreases the risk of arching your back. Try the leg raise, reverse crunch, and pelvic thrust.

• **Leg Raise.** Lie on your back with your hands under your lower back or buttocks for support until you have built up a good strength base. Raise your legs 6 inches off the floor and hold for a few seconds, while pressing your lower back into the floor. Raise your legs an additional 6 inches and hold. Finally, raise your legs another 6 inches and hold, before lowering your legs back to the initial position. Do not allow your abs to rest by dropping your feet all the way to the floor.

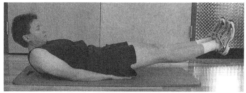

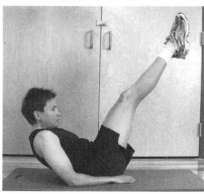

Keep your head off the floor for lower ab exercises. You may place your hands under your lower back and bend the legs slightly.

• **Reverse Crunch.** Lie on your back with your knees bent and your feet about an inch off the floor. Bring your pelvis and legs up until your knees are above your chest. Raise your pelvis a few inches off the floor. Lower your legs back to the starting position without touching your feet to the floor. This keeps constant tension on your abs. Repeat.

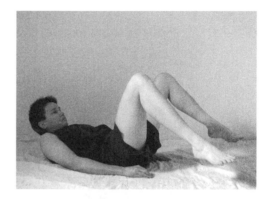

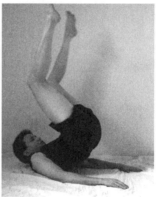

The reverse crunch is a good preparatory exercise for the pelvic thrust.

• **Pelvic Thrust.** If done with straight legs, this is a good ab exercise that requires quite a bit of strength. Start as you would with leg raises, but bring your legs all the way up until your feet are pointing toward the ceiling. Raise your pelvis a few inches off the floor by thrusting your feet vertically toward the ceiling. Keep your head off the floor. Lower your legs back to the starting position. Repeat.

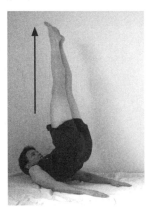

Your legs should be vertically straight. Do not allow them to tilt toward your head.

The obliques

The obliques twist the torso. Some believe that we can get rid of love handles by doing twisting exercises. But remember, love handles are excess fat, and in order to decrease fat, you must eat a leaner diet and fewer calories. For the purpose of this book, when training the obliques, you should focus on building strength, not on reducing fat. Try the trunk rotation, diagonal crunch, and side V-up.

• **Trunk Rotation.** Sit on the floor with your knees bent. If just starting out, have your partner hold your feet steady until you can do the exercise without a partner. Lean back to about 45 degrees and extend your arms straight in front of you. Clasp your hands together. Twist your body 90 degrees to the side. Pause for a second at full contraction. Repeat on the other side. To make the exercise more difficult, grab a set of dumbbells.

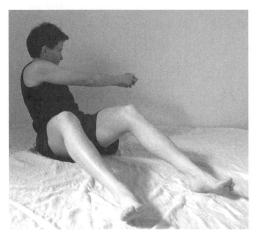

Make sure you maintain an incline in your upper body to the rear throughout the exercise.

• **Diagonal Crunch.** Lie on your back with your knees bent and your feet on the floor. Place one leg across the other. Place one hand behind your head. Reach with your opposite hand across your body toward your knee (left hand to right knee).

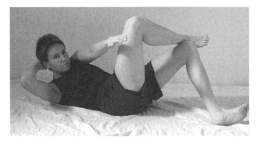

At full contraction, one shoulder should be off the floor.

• **Side V-Up.** Lie on your side with your top hand behind your head and your bottom hand on the floor for support. Keep a slight bend in your knees. Bring your lower and upper body together, until your body forms a V.

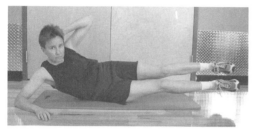

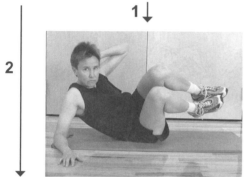

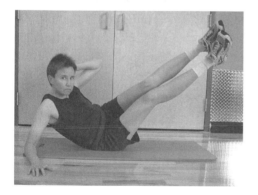

If you lack significant strength in your obliques, you can start with the modified version of the side V-up (1), before moving on to the full version (2).

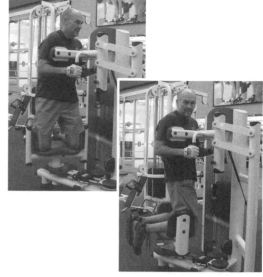

Try the reverse trunk twist on a machine. Your upper body remains stationary, while your lower body twists. This exercise works the entire midsection in addition to the obliques.

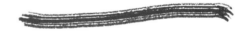

Ocean Swim

Remember the importance of training opposing muscle pairs to avoid muscle imbalance and maintain strength around your joints? Make sure you train your back along with your abdominals. For example, after you have completed a set of ab exercises, roll over on your belly and do a set of "ocean swim" back exercises. Pretend that you are swimming in the ocean, and every time you meet a wave, bob on this wave by raising your upper body as high as possible. Throughout the exercise, keep your arms extended forward, slightly to the side, or rested behind your head or back. Keep your thighs raised off the floor.

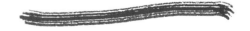

The upper abs

The upper abs are worked mainly through situps or crunches. Crunches are often more popular than full situps, because you use less of the hip flexors. Personally, I avoid taking an extreme position on this subject, and feel that the full situp has benefited me considerably. It's your choice. Keep in mind that a problem with the crunch is that it is easy to cheat by basically just nodding your head. If you do the crunch, you need to bring your shoulders and upper back off the floor, and avoid relaxing until you get to the end of your set. Try the bent leg crunch, vertical leg crunch, and stability ball crunch.

• **Bent Leg Crunch.** Lie on your back with your legs bent and your feet on the floor. Place your hands behind your head and press your lower back into the floor. This will tilt your pelvis toward your abdominal region. Raise your upper torso toward your knees. Limit the movement to about 30 degrees to avoid involving the hip flexors. Pause for a second at full contraction.

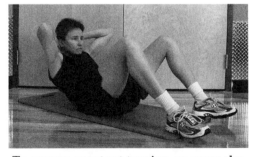

To ensure constant tension on your abs throughout the exercises, do not touch your shoulders to the floor when coming back to the starting position.

• **Vertical Leg Crunch.** Lie on your back with your legs extended vertically toward the ceiling. Place your hands behind your head and lift your upper torso toward your knees. Pause for a second at full contraction. Lower your upper body down, but do not touch your shoulders to the floor. Repeat.

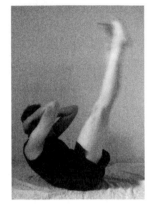

Make sure you lift your shoulders off the floor and not just nod your head.

• **Stability Ball Crunch.** Lie on your back on the stability ball with your feet flat on the floor. Place your hands behind your head. Lift your upper torso by contracting your abs. Remember, this exercise is more difficult because of the instability of the ball, and is also quite effective because of the 15 degrees of spinal extension. To make the exercise easier, place the ball under the upper part of your back; to make the exercise more difficult, place the ball under the lower part of your back. (see pg. 158)

Also work the upper abs against resistance on the crunch machine. The lower you place the pad, the more difficult the exercise is.

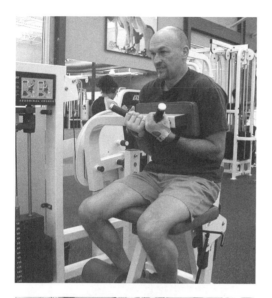

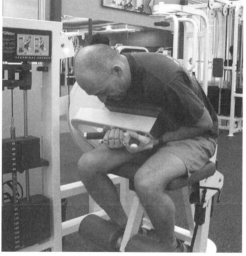

Plyometric Strengt

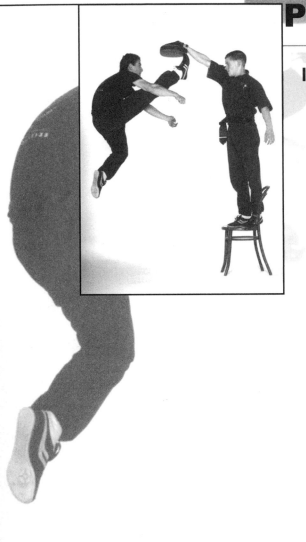

In this section:

- Power through plyometrics

- Explosiveness and inertia

- The stretch-shortening cycle

- When should you do plyometrics?

- Testing your explosive ability

- Lower body plyometric exercises

- Upper body plyometric exercises

Plyometric Strength

Think of plyometric strength as a measurement of your explosiveness, or how quickly your muscles can go from contraction to relaxation. Explosive power relates to force, and involves high intensity training and muscular contractions that use the stretch reflex. The stretch reflex is a protective reaction that causes muscles to contract, and can be triggered through moves that cause bouncing or overstretching.

Most of us agree that relaxation is important to speed, and that muscular contraction is important to power. But there is a fine line between tension and relaxation. If you are tense prior to throwing a strike, you will not have the necessary reaction time to take advantage of the opening in your opponent's defense; you will be too slow to be an efficient fighter. On the other hand, if you are too relaxed when landing the strike, you risk injury to the striking weapon and will be unable to produce enough power to do damage.

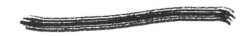

Benefits of Plyometrics

Plyometrics use gravity to store energy in the muscles before releasing that energy in the opposite direction. Explosive strength gives you the ability to accelerate your strikes suddenly, or to set your body in motion, stop motion, or change direction within a split second. Plyometric conditioning is also a good general strength and endurance builder.

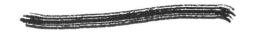

Power through plyometrics

Power is the rate of muscular force contraction over the range of motion in a specific time period. Power, in sports, is generally defined as the ability to produce force in a short period of time. Power is important in just about every sport I know of, even in sports that do not require you to hit your opponent. Power includes more than the ability to knock your opponent out. Power determines how fast you can swing a golf club or jump to slam-dunk a basketball. In martial arts, power allows you to throw your strikes and kicks faster or to close or widen a gap, placing yourself in a better position for dominating your opponent. Power has a lot to do with speed, so the faster you can set your body in motion, the more power you generally have. This can be translated into the power of a punch that is thrown with no telegraphing, or into the power of exploding your hips upward to unbalance an opponent who is straddling you on the ground.

Power relates to strength, and strength relates to speed and acceleration. The stronger you are, the easier it is to perform with power. This is true whether you initiate a move quickly, run or evade an attack, jump to perform a specific type of kick, throw a strike without telegraphing your move, or throw a weapon, such as a knife. Speed and acceleration are your keys to power. Sometimes, speed is consistent over a long period of time, as when running away or when throwing lengthy combinations, but more often, speed occurs in spurts. Power is therefore defined as your ability to use your force quickly. Bruce Lee said: "A powerful athlete is not a strong athlete, but one who can exert his strength quickly." This kind of explosive strength is achieved through plyometric training. Bench pressing 500 pounds is therefore not a correct definition of power for the purpose of martial arts.

Power relates to your timing and coordination. Sometimes, you must make split second decisions to throw or avoid a strike. If you don't, you will either get hit or fail to take advantage of the opening in your opponent's defense. Power in relation to position may be one of your greatest tactical advantages. Explosive power is also determined by your reaction time. You must perceive a need to move before you can respond to a stimulus. Training for power, thus training for speed and acceleration, might be the higher end objective in almost every athletic and competitive endeavor.

Impulse and Power

Impulse, or the change in momentum, is a physics concept that equals force X time. Impulse involves explosive force for the achievement of the greatest change in momentum in the shortest amount of time. In order to be powerful, you must have enough strength to control your own body mass in motion. Sometimes, you must also be strong enough to control your opponent's body mass in motion, for example, in grappling or close quarter arts. For a more detailed discussion of impulse, see *Fighting Science: The Laws of Physics for Martial Artists*, by Martina Sprague.

Explosiveness and inertia

Explosive speed relates to how quickly you can move your arms, feet, or body, and how quickly you can displace the mass of your opponent's body. Having explosive speed requires an ability to overcome inertia, or resistance to change in motion. The ability to overcome the inertia of your opponent's body, especially if he is heavier than you, is beneficial in such techniques as tackles, throws, takedowns, and in most grappling moves.

- Explosiveness allows you to read your opponent and time your block, counter-strike, or evasive move to his offense.

- Explosiveness allows you to move out of range or off the attack line, to reverse direction, and to place yourself in a superior position within range for a counter-attack. For example, if you choose to initiate with a tackle or throw, explosiveness allows you to drive forward with the tackle, or to pivot into position for the throw.

- Explosiveness allows you to start and stop movements in all directions, including lateral movements, twists, and pivots. It is not only the explosive start of a move that is important. Every sudden change in direction also requires a stop move.

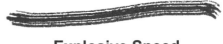

Explosive Speed

Explosive speed helps you dominate your opponent, react quickly to cues sent to you, increase your speed throughout a move, evade an attack, and time a counter-attack to the opening in his defense.

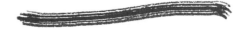

The stretch-shortening cycle

Remember how we talked about progressive overload in Chapter 5 on Understanding the Concepts? Muscles don't grow unless they are overloaded. When a task becomes too easy, you must make it difficult again. When you overload the muscle through plyometric exercise, you increase the explosive capability of the muscle. Using plyometric training along with regular strength training therefore helps you realize greater strength gains. "The main goal is to rapidly apply overload force to the muscles to improve speed strength. A plyometric exercise should be performed at a speed faster than you are capable of producing without some resistance." (www.building-muscle101. com)

Remember how we talked about concentric and eccentric muscle contractions in Chapter 2 on Muscle Anatomy? In concentric contractions, the muscle shortens; in eccentric contractions, the muscle lengthens, usually with the aid of gravity, producing force simultaneously, but without expending as much energy. This is why you are capable of doing a few extra reps eccentrically after you have exhausted the muscle concentrically. What is important here is that an eccentric contraction at high speed uses fast-twitch muscle fibers with a greater force production. This muscle lengthening eccentric contraction prior to the explosive concentric contraction is called the stretch-shortening cycle, and is the key element in plyometrics. Think of it as loading the muscle. During the eccentric phase, the muscle undergoes tension, or loading, where energy is stored within the muscle. Muscle elasticity, or how quickly the muscle can return to its original shape

when the load is released, creates force.

When you load the muscles quickly, you activate the stretch reflex, which causes powerful contraction of the muscles, or explosive power. In order to benefit from the stretch-shortening cycle, it must be performed rapidly. Think of it as a quick change of direction. Do not pause in the stretched position. **Be aware that large forces are produced in plyometrics, placing stress on your joints. Ease into plyometric training, listen to your body, and don't do plyometrics on several consecutive days.**

When should you do plyometrics?

Plyometric training is high intensity, so it is important to build a good strength base first. Body types and personal traits affect how well you can do plyometric exercises. For example, everybody doesn't have the same structural predisposition (body frame) for doing plyometric exercises without risking injury.

Plyometric exercises expose the muscles to repeated trauma, which can cause injuries or stress fractures in the affected body part. Sports science researchers also differ in opinion on the effectiveness of plyometrics, and some argue that the risks of injury far outweigh the potential benefits. "Plyometrics are controversial. Clearly, most of the support for plyometrics is based upon personal narratives and sketchy research. There is little scientific evidence that definitely proves plyometrics are productive." (A Practical Approach to Strength Training, Matt Brzycki)

In martial arts class, I often see the jumping jacks, pushups, ab work, stretches, plyometric dills, etc. done before class, with hardly any cool-down or stretching after class. I would recommend doing a light dynamic workout, such as shadow boxing before class, and the stretching and plyometric drills at the end of class, when your muscles are warm. When starting out, train in plyometrics for shorter intervals when you are rested. For example:

- Train in drills that last around 5-10 seconds.

- Every so often, train in longer explosive speed drills lasting up to 20 seconds.

- Decrease the rest period between drills to achieve a more fatigued state and greater stress.

- Consider the fact that you might have to use your quickness at the end of a match when you are fatigued.

When training in plyometrics, contact with the ground should be as short as possible between reps. For example, when doing pushups, your hands should leave the ground, and immediately push back off again upon completing a rep. When jumping, your feet should leave the ground, and immediately push back off again upon completing a rep. You can do plyometrics linearly, as when moving straight up, or laterally, as when moving to the side. Try a lateral plyometric jump by jumping from side-to-side, landing on one foot, remaining on that foot for about a second, and pushing off again and landing on the other foot. For starters, jump about three feet to the side. **Be careful with the landing and absorb the impact with your muscles, not with your joints.**

Testing your explosive ability

The type of muscle fiber called fast-twitch has the potential to develop sudden and explosive power. Those who are genetically predisposed to muscle dominated by fast-twitch fibers have an advantage over those genetically predisposed to muscle dominated by slow-twitch fibers. How do you know whether your plyometric training is making you stronger and more explosive? You know it by measuring the power of the concentric contraction of the muscle prior to starting your plyometric training, and again after you have trained for a while. For example, to test upper body plyometric strength, compare before and after results in the following exercises:

- How heavy a weight you can lift in the bench press

- How quickly you can lift the weight

- How hard you can hit a heavy bag

- How quickly you can set your strike in motion

- How high your hands come off the floor in a plyometric pushup

- How far you can throw a heavy object, for example, a 30-pound sandbag

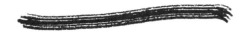

Plyometric Dodging Exercise

• Play a game of tag with your martial arts buddies in a fairly large area, for example, in your martial arts training hall.

• Depending on how quick you are, split up with one against three, four, or five opponents. Attempt to get through to the other side of the area without getting tagged.

• Try different variations, for example, four on two instead of four on one.

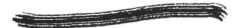

Lower body plyometric exercises

Lower body plyometrics involve a lot of jumping. Sprinting up hills or stairs are also good exercises for increasing your ability to accelerate. Work on quick starts and short sprint distances of 50-100 yards. Whether jumping or sprinting, push off with the ball of your rear foot rather than pulling forward with your lead foot. A common mistake is to treat the foot as a solid object. It is not, and sprint speed can be increased significantly by pushing with the ball of the foot rather than with the whole bottom of the foot. The harder you push, the longer your stride and the greater your speed. Compare this to throwing a strike. Your arm is not a rigid stick, and your fist either snaps closed or turns from vertical to horizontal at impact to increase the acceleration and penetration capabilities of the strike.

When working on quickness, start with your knees slightly bent to avoid using up time needlessly getting into position before you can execute your move. Speed and quickness drills should be multidirectional, requiring several start-stop moves and changes in direction. Start with 2-4 sets, 5 reps. Rest for 2 minutes between sets. Try these lower body plyometric exercises:

• **Two-Legged Vertical High Jump.** Jump as high as possible. Reach for a spot or mark on the wall.

• **Knees to Chest Jump.** Jump as high as you can, quickly bringing your knees to your chest. Touch your knees with your hands. Try to pause, or *hang*, for a second at the greatest height of the jump.

• **Jump Squat.** Start in the squat position and explode upward until your feet leave the floor. Land in the squat position and repeat.

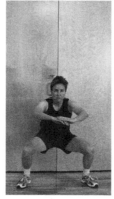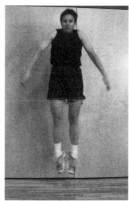

Jump squat, start with 2 sets, 5 reps.

• **Box Jump.** Jump up on an obstacle, landing on both feet simultaneously. Jump down backwards. Repeat. Start with a low obstacle, such as a low step-up aerobic bench. Increase the height as you get better. If using a chair for this, make sure a partner holds it steady to avoid injury.

• **Lateral Box Jump.** Jump from the side up on a low barrier, landing on both feet. Immediately jump down on the other side. Repeat in the other direction.

• **Two-Legged Lateral Jump Over Barrier.** Start with a low barrier, such as a step-up aerobic bench. Jump from left to right and back.

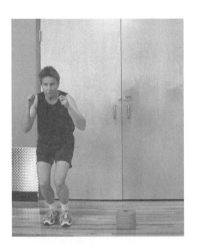

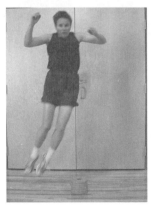

Two-legged lateral jump, start with 2 sets, 5 reps, alternate in each direction.

• **One-Legged Lateral Jump Over Barrier.** Same as two-legged jump, but start on your right foot, jump to the left and land on your left foot. Repeat in the other direction.

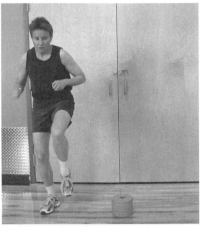

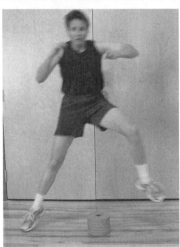

One-legged jump, start with 2 sets, 5 reps, alternate in each direction.

• **Stair Jump.** Jump up a stairway or bleachers, pushing off and landing on both feet simultaneously.

• **Two-Legged Long Jump.** Push off with both feet and jump as far forward as possible. Land on both feet and repeat.

• **One-Legged Long Jump.** Same as two-legged long jump, but alternate feet like a long stride. For example, push off with your right foot and land on your left foot. Immediately push off with your left foot and land on your right foot.

• **Power Skip.** Same as one-legged long jump, but strive for height simultaneously with distance.

• **Lunge Jump.** Stand in a right leg forward lunge. Jump and switch feet in the air, landing with your left leg forward.

Upper body plyometric exercises

Upper body plyometrics involve a lot of pushups and throwing of weighted objects, such as an 8-20 pound medicine ball. When starting with explosive strength pushups, lower yourself toward the floor and pause for a few seconds, then explode up in the pushup until your hands leave the floor. Start with 2-4 sets, 5 reps. Rest for 2 minutes between sets. Try these upper body plyometric exercises:

• **Plyometric Pushup.** Push off hard enough for your hands to leave the floor. As soon as your hands touch the floor, forcefully push back up again.

• **Alternating Wide/Narrow Pushup.** Push up from a wide hand position until your hands leave the floor and land in a narrow hand position. Push back up and land in a wide hand position. Keep alternating.

• **Obstacle Pushup.** Start with your hands narrowly spaced on the floor between two low obstacles, for example, between two weight stacks placed a little wider than shoulder-width apart. Push off and land with your hands widely spaced on top of the obstacles. Rebound back down on the floor. *Caution: Test the obstacles for stability before attempting this exercise.*

• **Clapping Pushup.** Add a handclap to each explosive pushup. This requires you to push off the floor hard enough to allow your hands to come together and clap prior to landing again.

• **Medicine Ball Upward Throw.** Kneel on the floor and hold the medicine ball at chest level. Keep your back straight. Throw the ball at a diagonal angle upward and forward while extending your upper body. It is acceptable to fall forward and catch yourself on your hands.

• **Medicine Ball Drop and Throwback.** Lie on the floor and catch a medicine ball that your partner drops toward your chest. Immediately throw it back.

• **Medicine Ball Situp and Throw.** Lie on the floor and throw the medicine ball to your partner as you sit up. Catch the ball when your partner throws it back to you and immediately lie back down on the floor. Repeat.

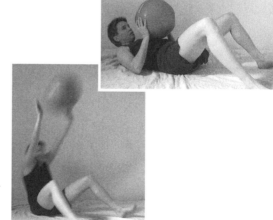

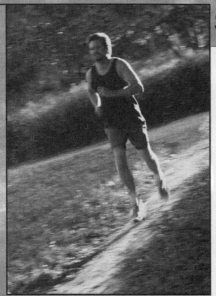

Cardiovascular Strength Endurance

In this section:

- How fast does your heart beat?

- Transfer of skill

- Cardio through strength training

- Anaerobic training

- Cardio or weight-lifting first?

- High intensity interval training

- Chase the rabbit, eat the dirt

Cardiovascular Strength Endurance

How fast does your heart beat?

The focus of this book is on developing muscular strength, but since the martial arts require a combination of muscular strength and cardiovascular fitness, I want to devote at least one chapter to strengthening the heart and relating it to muscular strength.

To improve cardiovascular endurance, you need to exercise your heart a minimum of 2 days per week, but 3-5 days is recommended. A good strength program is built around intensity of training, and so is a good cardiovascular program. For example, running intermingled with sprints builds your cardiovascular fitness faster than walking. Time or duration is also important. If you have the choice of quick walking for 30 minutes or intense sprints for 5 minutes, the longer time of walking will benefit you more in cardiovascular terms. In general, your cardio program should last no less than 20 minutes of sustained effort, with a target intensity of 70-80 percent of your maximum heart rate according to age, and up to 90-100 percent for optimal conditioning.

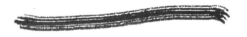

Think About This

Your cardio program should include weight lifting or muscular strength training. If you train only in cardiovascular fitness, you will not develop any significant muscle growth. In fact, you might lose muscle mass. Keep your goals in mind when designing your strength and cardio program.

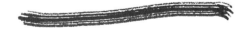

When you are in great cardiovascular shape, your heart rate will slow down sometimes to only 45 beats per minute at rest. This slower heart rate makes each beat more efficient for pumping the blood through the body. This efficiency allows you to work at a higher intensity for a longer duration of time, because you don't have to expend as much energy as a person of lesser conditioning. Getting winded in sparring is extremely debilitating. If you have experienced it in competition, you know what I'm talking about. If you enter a sparring match, and you know you have a strong heart, your confidence grows, because you know that you can pick up the pace, overwhelm your opponent, and still outlast him.

How fast our hearts beat is inversely related to our physical size. A big person has a slower heartbeat than a small person. This is why most women have slightly faster resting heart rates than most men – not because they are women, but because they are smaller in size and therefore have smaller hearts. In general, "women's hearts beat 6-8 times per minute faster than those of men." (A Practical Approach to Strength Training, Matt Brzycki) Compare this to one of the smaller creatures of the world – the hummingbird: "A resting hummingbird takes 250 breaths per minute (4 times a second). A (heart) rate of 1260 beats per minute has been measured (20 times that of a human heart). The hummingbird family contains the smallest of all birds; many species are less than 8 cm in overall length. The smallest species is the bee hummingbird of Cuba. Its males are slightly smaller than females, being about 5.5 cm long, and weighing only 1.95 grams, which is just a tiny fraction of the weight of a first-class letter." (Colibri Pro Development AB, www.colibri.se)

Your target heart rate when exercising is between 70 and 80 percent of your maximum heart rate, and decreases with age. As a guideline:

At age 20, your target heart rate is 120-170 beats per minute

At age 30, your target heart rate is 114-162 beats per minute.

At age 40, your target heart rate is 108-153 beats per minute.

At age 50, your target heart rate is 102-145 beats per minute.

At age 60, your target heart rate is 96-136 beats per minute.

At age 70, your target heart rate is 90-128 beats per minute.

As you can see, there is a wide range of acceptable heart rates for each age group. (WebMD Medical Reference in collaboration with the Cleveland Clinic)

Transfer of skill

Skill is increased when you practice your martial art repeatedly. But you must do exercises that are transferable. Many skills are not transferable. For example, you might have the cardiovascular endurance to run 10 miles, but not the endurance to spar 10 rounds. What this means is that you cannot necessarily gain the endurance you need for kickboxing by doing a lot of running. I still recommend running as a supplementary exercise, because it is one of the better cardio activities that also strengthens your legs and helps bring variety to your workout.

When running for the purpose of strengthening the heart and gaining transferable skills, you must run with intent. Jogging doesn't qualify. It is better to do a fast-stride walk than a jog, because a stride also gives you speed and extension in the hips, which jogging doesn't provide. The ability to do a long stride can carry over into a martial arts skill, for example, a shuffle-step used to move in on an opponent. Do several running variations:

• Run at an even and reasonably fast pace, for example, a 9-minute mile pace.

• Do several shorter sprints, for example, sprint 100 yards and walk back. Repeat.

• Combine walking, striding, running, and sprinting in 100-yard increments.

• Accelerate and decelerate several times throughout a 1-mile run.

• Run hills with short segments of different inclines.

Cardio through strength training

An intense and properly conducted training program builds both your muscular strength and your cardiovascular fitness. Although your focus is on muscular strength when lifting weights, the cardio system benefits, in some instances more than if you go running, cycling, or do aerobics. An added benefit is that weight training may also be gentler on your joints than a lot of running or aerobics. "Most have never heard that great benefits to the cardiovascular system, commonly referred to as aerobic fitness, can be had through a program of high-intensity strength training with no additional steady-state activity." (High Intensity Strength Training: More Aerobic Than "Aerobics," by Master Instructor Greg Anderson at Ideal Exercise in Seattle)

High intensity means hard work. You increase the intensity by:

- Increasing the resistance (the load)

- Decreasing the rest between sets

The reason strength training benefits the heart is because, when you strength-train at high intensity, there is an increase in muscular activity. Increased muscular activity places demands on the heart. As a result, you will up your performance in cardio activities. However, the reverse is not true: A good heart does not necessarily give you better muscular strength.

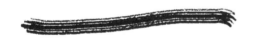

Transfer of Muscular Strength

If you want to train the cardiovascular system, high intensity strength training is an effective way to help you achieve cardiovascular fitness. The muscular strength you gain is also easily transferable to different types of activities in the martial arts. Do not neglect training your muscles at the expense of training your heart.

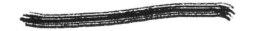

The benefit of weight training for cardiovascular fitness was researched and written about as early as 1976, in a project termed "Project Total Conditioning," conducted at the United States Military Academy at West Point, by James A. Peterson, Ph.D. The paper was presented to the Pre-Montreal Olympic Conference of the International Congress of Physical Activity Science, Quebec City, Canada, July 15, 1976: " . . . by maintaining the intensity of the training at a high level, substantial improvement was achieved in both the level of muscular fitness and the cardiovascular condition . . . these results are contrary to the traditional viewpoint that weight training does not affect the cardiovascular efficiency of the individual trainee . . . a high intensity workout of relatively short duration resulted in improvement in more than merely the level of muscular fitness . . ."

So how much can you improve your cardiovascular fitness through strength training? In the early 1970's, Arthur Jones, the inventor of the Nautilus exercise machines, claimed that you could reach greater results with short and infrequent routines, as opposed to long hours each day. A study was conducted at the West Point Military Academy, with the following passage excerpted from Flexibility and Metabolic Condition, by Arthur Jones: "In a period of less than six weeks, a group of 19 football players increased their strength by an average of approximately 60 percent . . . an equally significant improvement in cardiovascular endurance was produced simultaneously . . . as a result of the same very brief training program that produced the spectacular strength increases."

In a transcript from The Medicine Man Television Program, Arthur Jones goes on to say: "Any, ANY, result that can be produced by any amount of running can be duplicated and surpassed by the proper use of weight lifting for cardiovascular benefits." Remember, though, in order to achieve results, you must use a proper program and train with intent. Any program, not properly used, will yield low results.

The good part about all of this is that you no longer need to think of muscular strength and cardio fitness separately. For example, you don't have to go and run 3 miles, and then go to the gym and lift weights (although you can for variation). Weight lifting alone, as long as it is done at high intensity, benefits your heart. Think about this: If you can increase muscular strength while simultaneously increasing your cardiovascular fitness . . . that's what I call "catching two flies with one swat." Combining training regimens saves you time, allowing you to accomplish more.

Aerobics and Weight Loss

If your goal is to lose weight by losing fat, it helps to know that one pound of fat can fuel the average person's body for approximately 10 hours of activity. Thus, if you run a marathon (26 miles), you will probably lose no more than half a pound of weight, at the most. Any additional loss is most likely water weight, which you will regain as soon as you replace the fluid loss. Aerobic activity is therefore not the greatest form of weight loss activity. In contrast, an additional pound of muscle allows you to consume approximately 100 additional calories per day, just to sustain that muscle. So muscular strength training is a more efficient way of achieving weight loss than is aerobic training.

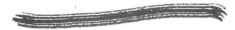

A note about anaerobic training

We have now established that you can get a great deal of cardiovascular benefit from high intensity strength training, but you must maintain the intensity during the workout and limit the amount of rest between sets. When you give it some thought you will see that many martial arts rely on cardiovascular capacity and muscular strength at the same time. For example, jump kicks or combination kicks, flurries of punches, quick footwork, intense sparring, and throws and grappling. If you want to improve cardio performance through high intensity training, you must push your training up a notch. This is why sprinting, or at least running at a good pace, is recommended over jogging. But you must also keep in mind that the higher intensity training has a greater injury rate associated with it, such as pulled muscles or sprained ankles.

In contrast to aerobic exercise, which means "with oxygen," *anaerobic* exercise, which means "without oxygen," includes any training that requires an all-out effort followed by a period of partial rest. In anaerobic training, the muscles rely on stored reserves of fuel. Since the reserve fuel (the small amount of oxygen found in the muscle tissue) is quickly used up, the body goes into oxygen debt and is unable to continue at high intensity for longer than approximately one minute; however, this time can be improved upon with training. The good part about anaerobic training is that it develops strength also during the recovery process, when the body releases a growth hormone to the muscles. Anaerobic exercises include sprints (could be while running, cycling, swimming, sparring, or grappling), and weight and resistance training.

Cardio or weight-lifting first?

If you choose to include specific cardio exercises in your strength program, you can do your cardio training on the same days you do your strength training, or on the in-between days. Same day cardio might be more efficient, because it allows you to recover completely on your in-between days, but both choices are acceptable. Time of day is of little importance. You often hear stories of professional boxers getting up and running in pre-dawn at four o'clock in the morning. This has more to do with discipline and the feeling that you are a step ahead of your competition, than with any actual aerobic benefits. If you are a morning person, do your cardio in the morning. If you are an evening person, do your cardio in the evening. Whatever fits your schedule is good.

If you do cardio and strength training on the same day, which should you do first? I have been unable to find a single answer to this question. "If you're reasonably fit, I suggest you do 15-20 minutes of aerobics first, followed by 10 minutes of mid-section exercise, and finish up, unpressured and focused, with your weight routine. Less fit people prefer to warm up only for 5 minutes before weight training in order to conserve energy, doing the remainder of their cardio upon completion. Some reserve their cardio for the end of their workout, aiming to burn their excess calories. There are good arguments for all. You choose as you become familiar with your training." (www.bodybuilding.com)

High intensity interval training

You might be lifting weights regularly several times a week, but when it is time to spar, you are wheezing from oxygen deprivation halfway through the first round. If you want to improve your cardiovascular endurance, you must push yourself and exercise beyond what is comfortable. Interval training incorporates higher intensity exercise with lower intensity exercise.

Aerobics and cardio are not the same, but the uneducated often use these words interchangeably. Aerobics is low intensity training performed for a longer duration, for example, for 40 minutes in an aerobic studio. Your body gets used to this and, although you have been going to aerobic class for years, you see no improvement in your endurance. Cardio is of higher intensity and of shorter duration, and might be performed for only 15-20 minutes at a time. Cardio can be taken up to the level of high intensity. If you add intervals, with a short period of exercise followed by a short period of rest, you will have a highly effective program for building muscle mass, strength, endurance, and aerobic capacity. Here is how to optimize your aerobic/cardio training:

High Intensity Intervals

Do a 5-minute warm-up and some light stretching prior to starting the interval training. During the intervals, your heart rate should reach 90-95 percent of your maximum heart rate. When first starting out, limit the high intensity training to 5 minutes. As you get stronger, increase to

15 minutes. Cool down and stretch after finishing.

Option 1: Sprint up a hill (30 seconds). Walk down (2 minutes). Repeat.

Option 2: Punch a heavy bag consistently and as fast as you can (20 seconds). Shadow box or do a martial arts form (30 seconds). Repeat.

Option 3: Run at a steady 9-minute mile pace on the treadmill (2 minutes). Drop down for 20 pushups. Repeat.

Option 4: Jump rope as fast as you can (30 seconds). Jump at half-speed (1 minute). Repeat.

Option 5: Do 10 squat thrusts as fast and high as you can. Do 20 jumping jacks at normal speed. Repeat.

Hint: If you are untrained, take a few weeks to pre-condition yourself for the interval training by doing 5 minutes of walking and 5 minutes of running for 20-30 minutes. Or do 1 minute of walking and 1 minute of running for 20 minutes.

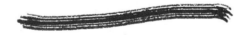

Extra Edge

Do a 1-mile timed run for cool down. Make sure you improve on your time every few weeks. For example, start at a 12-minute mile pace and work up to a 9-minute mile pace.

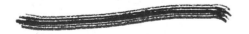

Now that you are on your way toward realizing significant improvements in cardiovascular fitness, try the Navy Seal student preparation workout. The Navy Seals are the most prestigious elite of all, and if you can get through just the first week of their grueling 18-week preparatory training program, I applaud you:

<u>Navy Seal Workout Week One</u>

(www.navyseals.com)

Running: 2 miles, 8.5-min mile pace (Mon/Wed/Fri)

Pushups: 4 sets of 15 pushups (Mon/Wed/Fri)

Situps: 4 sets of 20 situps (Mon/Wed/Fri)

Pull-ups: 3 sets of 3 pull-ups (Mon/Wed/Fri)

Swimming: Swim continuously for 15 minutes (4-5 days/week)

Chase the Rabbit, Eat the Dirt

Now that you have built some strength and endurance and know what I'm talking about, let's finish every workout with my favorite high intensity training exercise, called "chase the rabbit, eat the dirt." Start by working each segment for approximately 20 seconds, and at the highest intensity speed you can muster.

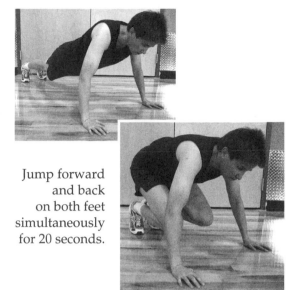

Jump forward and back on both feet simultaneously for 20 seconds.

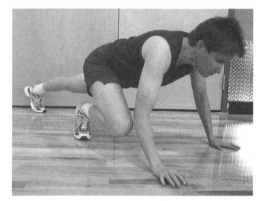

Get down on all four and alternate your feet forward and back as fast as you can for 20 seconds.

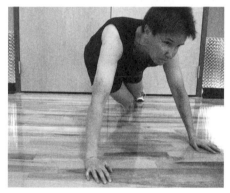

Go down the ski hill as fast as you can for 20 seconds.

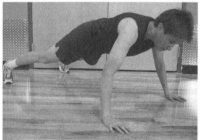

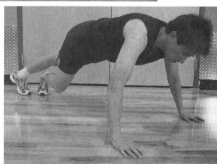

Criss-cross your feet behind you as fast as you can for 20 seconds.

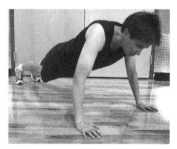

Eat the dirt 10 times. Repeat the cycle 2 more times.

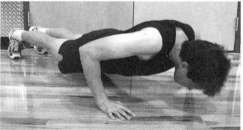

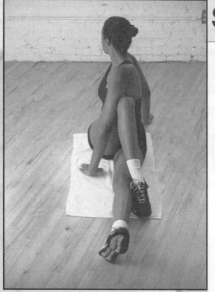

Flexibility and Strength

In this section:

- Flexibility defined

- Is stretching worth your time?

- Types of stretches

- How much should you stretch?

- Stretching for warm-up

- Genetics and stretching

- Functional flexibility

Flexibility and Strength

Everybody knows the martial arts require great flexibility. In fact, when people find out I'm a martial artist, the first question they ask (after they have asked if I'm a black belt) is if I can do full splits or kick to the head. But those who have studied the arts for some time know that kicking to the head is not an absolute necessity. In fact, many arts require only low kicks to the legs, and the grappling or throwing arts may not require kicks at all. As you grow older, or if you start in the arts at an advanced age, you may not be able to throw high kicks. Your ability to kick high is not the only determinant of whether or not you can become a successful fighter.

The question, then, is not necessarily whether flexibility is important, but rather how important it is. How do we define flexibility, and what will it do for you? Will it make you more efficient? Less prone to injury? How do we know? Rather than asking whether stretching helps prevent injury, it might be better asking, how does stretching benefit you, and in what situations?

Since this book is about strength and not flexibility, we need to find a way to relate flexibility to strength and look at it from that perspective. Being flexible can help you improve speed and power. "Increased flexibility, when married to a progressive strength-training program, will expand the distance over which the muscle force is applied. For example, if a sprinter can improve his stride length via enhanced flexibility, his force application now covers a greater distance, which should result in augmented power and speed." (Flexible Perspectives on Stretching, Ken Mannie, www.naturalstrength.com) This can be verified through the Power Formula in physics:

Power = work / time
Work = force X distance

so if you make the substitution:

Power = force X distance / time

For more in-depth discussions of power, see *Fighting Science: The Laws of Physics for Martial Artists*, by Martina Sprague.

Flexibility defined

Martial arts fitness requires a combination of strength, endurance, and flexibility. Although your body is comprised of many separate "units," such as your legs, arms, trunk, and neck, you must look at your body as a whole; you can't treat just one unit and expect to achieve fitness or efficiency in athletics. Good flexibility results in:

- Full range of motion
- Economy of motion
- Less muscular effort

Flexibility is a highly individual matter. Some people are unable to improve their flexibility in a specific joint, because the joint is limited by its skeletal structure rather than by the muscles and tendons. A person can also have different levels of flexibility in different joints of his body. For example, he might have flexible arms and wrists, but less flexible legs. When working to increase your flexibility, remember that a joint has two sides, and that you must exercise both sides to avoid limiting your flexibility based on the ability of the less flexible side of the joint.

Training Tip

When using weight training to enhance flexibility, use full range of motion. Do not cheat by moving the weight through a limited distance.

Is stretching worth your time?

Being flexible allows you to perform faster and stronger moves while maintaining your balance. "An athlete with flexibility generates acceleration over a greater range of motion, thereby increasing speed." (High-Performance Sports Conditioning, Bill Foran) In the martial arts, especially if you study a mixed art, you need to switch positions often, going from standing, to kneeling, to prone, or to supine. Being flexible helps you switch positions with greater ease, whether for offense or defense, and re-establish a superior position in relation to your opponent. Switching positions with ease involves the coordination of muscles, which is enhanced through flexibility. The importance of flexibility seems pretty obvious. But in March of 2004, the CDC (Centers for Disease Control) published the results of a study that hit me square in the face: *Stretching doesn't prevent injuries.*

The report was published in the March 2004 issue of the American College of Sports Medicine Journal. Stephen B. Thacker,

director of the epidemiology program office at the Centers for Disease Control and Prevention said that they could not find a benefit, and that athletes who stretch might feel more limber, but they shouldn't count on stretching to keep them healthy: "The use of stretching primarily as a way to prevent sports injury has been based on intuition and observation rather than scientific evidence," said lead researcher Stephen B. Thacker, M.D. "The best advice is to include a combination of warm-up, strength training, plyometrics and balance exercises to lessen injury risks."

The report goes on to say: "While the evidence does show that stretching is important in increasing muscle and joint flexibility, in most cases researchers found little-to-no relationship between stretching and injuries or post-exercise pain." Thacker also found that, "Most injuries occur during muscle contractions within the normal range of joint motion anyway, so it's unclear how increasing the range of motion through stretching would decrease injury risk." A muscle pull most often results from a muscle that isn't prepared to work in its normal range of motion, rather than in a muscle that hasn't been stretched.

Does this mean that we should bag stretching? I feel this would be disastrous, but you should put it in perspective. Whether or not stretching directly helps prevent injuries, stretching still increases the blood flow to the muscles and helps ready your body for training. Flexibility is still an element of fitness. Being limber and ready to respond to sudden changes, such as what one might experience when attacking or defending in the martial arts, also affects your ability to keep your balance. I'm sure nobody disputes that being stretched out and limber helps you perform your moves with greater ease. My opinion is that even if stretching doesn't prevent injuries, it is still beneficial to the martial artist. It is difficult to perform your art when your body is stiff. Depending on your art and goals, being limber might also improve performance, for example, in musical forms competition or gymnastic type moves that require the performance of difficult acrobatic maneuvers. Overall, I believe it would be a mistake to eliminate stretching and flexibility exercises from your strength training or martial arts program.

In the end, when determining whether stretching is worth your time, you might want to consider the specific requirements of your sport. The CDC found that, "People such as gymnasts and dancers might be the exceptions, because their activities require great flexibility," while Mike Bracko, director of the Institute for Hockey Research in Calgary, Alberta, said, "We have done some work with hockey players showing flexibility is not an important variable." Bracko goes on to say that a tear typically happens when a muscle has to react suddenly to control an athlete's movement, which suggests that it is the sudden or unexpected movement we need to be concerned with regarding injury prevention, and not how flexible a muscle is or how far it can stretch. (The Associated Press, 2004)

Flexibility and Strength

A study on workplace stretching programs found that strength training combined with stretching makes a person more limber: "Flexibility improved in those who performed strength training and stretching, but not in those who performed only strengthening exercises. Also, stretching combined with strength training resulted in higher percentage increases in static and dynamic strength than did strength training alone." (University of Oregon, Labor Education and Research Center)

Types of stretches

Flexibility can be broken down into static and dynamic. You can think of static flexibility as the range of motion of a joint, and dynamic flexibility as the ease with which you can move the joint through its range of motion. There are several different types of stretches:

• **Proprioceptive Neuromuscular Facilitation (PNF)** combines muscle contraction and relaxation. For example, contract the muscle for 15-20 seconds, relax, and then stretch. This type of stretch has shown to have the greatest effect. Try this: Stand with your back to a wall and have your partner raise your leg straight up in front of you. Push your heel into the palm of your partner's hand while he provides resistance. When you relax, your partner should be able to raise your leg slightly higher than prior to the stretch.

• **Static stretches** with no movement of the muscle during the stretch. For example, your partner raises your leg until you feel the stretch, and holds your leg steady for 15-20 seconds. This type of stretch is effective, but takes second place to the PNF stretch. When doing static stretches, you might reach full range of motion of the muscle, but since the muscle is held stationary and sports are about moving, this type of stretch does not contribute directly to the movement you need in your sport. The static stretch might be most beneficial after a training session, when your muscles are already warm and you can ease into the stretch.

• **Isometric stretches or contractions** with no change in the length of the muscle have been found to be more effective than static stretches (iso = equal, isometric = equal metric or equal length). Isometric contraction means that there is tensing of the stretched muscle; you contract the muscle while it is being stretched. For example, rather than raising your leg as high as it goes and simply holding it there, when you reach maximum height, you contract your hamstring against the resistance of your partner's hand. Since your partner is providing resistance, your hamstring is unable to bend your leg, yet the muscle still contracts. When working isometric stretches, you can also work without a partner and provide resistance through the use of a wall, table, windowsill, or with your own limbs, depending on which muscle group you are stretching. For example, an isometric triceps stretch can be done by bending your arm behind your neck (elbow pointed toward the ceiling) and using your opposite hand to provide resistance while you tense the triceps muscle. A calf stretch can be done by sitting on the floor with your leg extended in front of you. Hold on to the ball of your foot while tensing your calf in an attempt to straighten your foot against the resistance of your hand. Hold each stretch for 15-20 seconds, then relax for 20 seconds, and repeat.

• **Ballistic stretches**, where you bounce the muscle during the stretch. This type of stretch has shown a higher injury rate and should therefore be avoided. A tear typically happens when a muscle has to react suddenly to unexpected movement. However, my personal experience is that some light "pulsing" while stretching is beneficial. Also, what I call movement stretches or dynamic stretches, which include shadow boxing, arm/leg/trunk rotations, etc. are more efficient than static stretches, and might help loosen your joints quicker.

How much should you stretch?

Next question is, how much time should one devote to stretching prior to or after exercise? How many repetitions constitute a good stretching program?

Not stretching at all may be detrimental, while stretching for two hours a day may not be cost/benefit effective, since you are taking time away from other forms of training that may benefit you more. When deciding on a stretching program, first define your objective clearly. Is it injury prevention? Flexibility/ease of movement? Strength or balance related? Also do a cost/risk/benefit analysis. What is the real value of stretching for your particular sport/martial art? At what point does the price become greater than the value? How much you stretch depends on the needs of your art.

A common fear is that strength training will make you muscle bound and reduce your flexibility. This is an outdated concern and has not been found to be true. You should not be afraid to lose flexibility simply because you lift weights. The greatest threat to flexibility is a general slowing down and lack of movement.

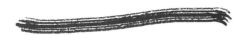

The Old Age Myth

Although a contributing factor to flexibility loss is old age, the main reason older people lose flexibility is not because their tissues get less elastic, but because older people are generally less active. The best way to maintain flexibility is to remain active, especially into old age. Disuse of muscles results in muscle atrophy and flexibility loss.

Stretching for warm-up

The martial arts require many, diverse, and quick moves, and stretching is often used as a warm-up activity. Warming up facilitates blood flow throughout the muscles and raises the body temperature. But studies about the importance of warm-up are somewhat inconclusive. Some say you will perform better if you warm up prior to martial arts practice; others say it makes no difference whether you warm up or not. My opinion is that at least some form of warm-up helps ready your body for training. I am in favor of a light dynamic or "moving" warm-up, consisting of light shadow boxing and dynamic stretches. In other words, this is not the time you want to sit in the splits and meditate.

When warming up, think about what your martial arts workout entails. Since the martial arts generally require large and diverse movements, the best way to ready your body is by doing exercises that mimic the martial arts; in other words, moving exercises. The warm-up should prepare you to move the way you are to move in your sport. If your martial art session is to include specific exercises, such as high kicks or joint locking techniques, you might want to include specific warm-up stretches for those muscle groups and joints. For example, stretching the hips and hamstrings is important if you are to do high kicks. A good dynamic warm-up for the legs is the lunge. Do the lunge across the room a number of times to stretch the hip and leg. Lateral lunges and hip rotations are also good exercises that take the legs through full range of motion. If you are to engage in joint locking techniques, stretching the shoulders, wrists, and fingers is important. However, spending time on warming up your hands is less valuable if today's workout is to focus only on kicks. I'm not saying that a total body warm-up is a bad idea, but if your time is limited, you should focus on warming up those muscles that are to be used specifically in your workout.

So if it is a good idea to stretch and warm up prior to martial arts training, is it also a good idea to do so prior to lifting weights? If you strength train in a controlled manner, there is generally no need to stretch or warm up prior to starting your weight lifting routine. However, there are differences of opinion here as well. "A warm-up is almost universally used at the beginning of an exercise or activity session to improve performance and prevent injury. The theory behind warm-ups is that muscular contractions are dependent on temperature. Because increased muscle temperature improves work capacity and a warm-up increases muscle temperature, it is assumed that warming up is necessary." (www.askmen.com)

Genetics and stretching

Just as genetics play a role in strength building, genetics also play a role in flexibility. Some people are just more natural when it comes to building strength or flexibility and, although most of us can improve on our current condition, we are not all capable of reaching equal results. If you were born with unfavorable genetics, rather than getting hung up on what you cannot do, turn your focus on what you can do and what types of flexibility benefit you the most. The flexibility that is important is that which allows you to do the techniques required for your art with ease. For example, being able to do full splits is not necessarily important, and may not even be attainable, no matter how much you train.

One of the problems is that in the martial arts we often equate flexibility only to the legs, without considering the arms, shoulders, neck, or body. We also make certain assumptions that may not be true. For example, I have heard it stated that women are more flexible than men, and that women can do splits, toe touches, and butterfly stretches easier than men. But before jumping on the bandwagon and assuming that women are more flexible than men, examine the general build of the female body and compare it to that of the male body. In general (not always), it can be said that women are shorter/smaller than men. Having short legs makes it easier to touch your toes, because you have a shorter distance to reach when bending over. This might create the visual illusion that you are more flexible.

Your flexibility potential is determined by your bones, muscles, tendons, ligaments, and skin. How flexible you are or can become varies greatly between individuals and depends on several factors, for example, the range of motion of your joints. If you run an experiment by randomly choosing a group of 100 women and a group of 100 men, you are likely to find greater variations in flexibility within a particular group than between groups. For example, the range of flexibility between individuals in the female group will be greater than the difference in average flexibility between the male and the female group. You can also have different degrees of flexibility in different joints. Thus, it is possible to have flexible hips but less flexible shoulders.

As of the writing of this book, I have trained in the martial arts for 18 years. I have always desired the ability to do full splits, but even with 18 years of training, I have seen virtually no improvement in my flexibility as far as the splits go. In fact, while other people say they feel the stretch along the inside thigh, I feel pain in my hip joint on the outside of my leg/butt. Stretching specialists tell you to do a simple test to determine whether you have the potential to achieve full splits: Stand on one leg and place your other leg straight out to the side with your foot on top of the back of a chair. Since the muscles don't cross from one leg to the other, if you can do this, then you also have the potential to achieve full splits. I fail this test. I can do it with the leg in the forward or back position, but not in the side position, which results in a tilt of my upper body to the side. I haven't had it verified medically, but my belief is that my limitation is due to deep hip sockets. In other words, it is a skeletal limitation, and not a muscular one. This is therefore an area that I cannot train efficiently.

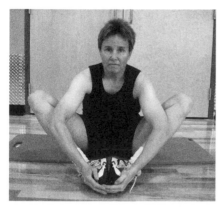

Because of the construction of my hips, I am unable to do a good butterfly stretch or split. While most people can place their knees completely on the floor (after some warm-up or stretching), my knees are at a greater than 45-degree angle. In other words, I can't even achieve half of the full butterfly position. This is after 18 years of training! My mom, who was a gymnast, is built the same way.

Note that if your bones are the limiting factor to movement, there is less you can do for further improvement. If you are not flexible enough to perform a required move, your body might compensate for it in other ways that are not anatomically efficient or that might result in injury, for example, by arching your back when throwing a high kick.

Functional flexibility

Many martial artists feel that flexibility in the legs is important so that they can achieve high kicks, but what about arm and shoulder flexibility, or trunk flexibility? What about flexibility to move with the forces (stance flexibility)? A flexible athlete can maintain balance easier, shift position quicker, use better technique with greater ease, and generally start and stop movement

faster. When stretching for sports, strive to develop range of motion in several planes and include the functional movement you are trying to achieve. You do this through dynamic (moving) stretches, such as lunges and arm and trunk rotations. In other words, sitting on the floor and stretching each leg singularly while holding the stretch is not the best way.

Depending on the requirements of your art, a greater degree of flexibility may be needed in some joints than in others. If your art relies mainly on grappling moves and low kicks, upper body and arm/wrist flexibility might be more important than hip flexibility. If your art requires mainly high kicks to score on your opponent, the opposite is true.

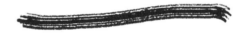

The Meaning of Functional Flexibility

Although the study performed by the CDC found that stretching does not make you more or less likely to suffer injuries, such as a pulled muscle, and that injuries typically happen within the muscle's normal range of motion, we must still recognize that lack of stretching decreases flexibility. Being flexible should not be seen as an end in itself. Although you might think that full splits look impressive, it is functional flexibility that enhances performance. Ask yourself in what ways your flexibility makes you better. It is not always as obvious as saying, "It helps me kick higher."

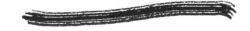

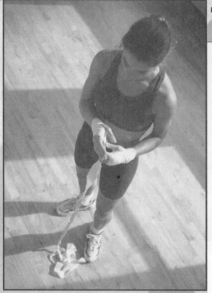

Women's Strength Training

In this section:

- **Warning for women**

- **The argument against strength training**

- **Gender difference**

- **Absolute strength comparisons fail**

Women's Strength Training

Who needs muscles? I recently heard a female martial artist say: "In jiu-jitsu, you don't need a lot of strength to execute techniques." Why is it that men fighting men realize the importance of strength training, and women fighting men think they don't have to strength train? This is the wrong attitude. Sure, anytime you can go against your opponent's weaknesses, such as his joints or his eyes, you need less strength than if you try to outbox him. However, these are ideal situations, and reality doesn't always strike that way.

Let's say that you are a female jiu-jitsu practitioner competing against another female jiu-jitsu practitioner. First, chances are you have both studied the same techniques and concepts. You can therefore predict your opponent's techniques, and she can predict yours. Second, you are most likely similar in build, size, and strength, so maybe you don't need a lot of strength to defeat your opponent.

Now, let's say that you are a female jiu-jitsu practitioner fighting a much bigger male, a karate guy, in fact, who doesn't know a thing about grappling. The fight goes to the ground, and you have all the technique advantages. The only problem is that your opponent has hands and forearms three times the size of yours. If this man has just a tiny bit of bend in his arm when you try to execute that armbar, he might defeat you solely based on his superior strength. Although your techniques are good under ideal conditions, if you lack strength against an opponent significantly bigger than you, your techniques become defeat-able. Good technique is no substitute for strength.

Warning for women

When asked how I feel I have been treated as a female martial artist in a male dominated environment, I say that there really haven't been any problems worth discussing. My opinion is that women are mostly responsible for the success or failure of their own journey. Sure, many women have not been brought up in a sports competitive environment, and have been conditioned to believe that it is okay for women to be ranked on the second rung of the athletic ladder. This includes traits such as strength, aggressiveness, courage, and independence. Some reconditioning might therefore be needed to lessen the emotional gap between those who see themselves purely as athletes, and those who see themselves as *female* or *male* athletes.

Women as a group are often judged on the performance of a few women who did not rise to the task, and not on their individual performances. You, as a woman, need to realize that your individual performance has nothing to do with what other women have done or not done in the past. You are your own boss on how far you want to go. If you remain physically unfit or fail to achieve competitive strength, it is primarily your own fault, and not the fault of the male population or other women's under-achievements. The perspective we will use when approaching the subject of women's strength training is that women's lack of physical strength and fitness has nothing to do with what men (or women, friends, parents) tell women they can or cannot do, and everything to do with what women tell themselves they can or cannot do. Start by taking full responsibility for your training and avoiding excuses such as, "women haven't had the same opportunities as men, girls are not encouraged to be aggressive or strong, women are genetically different from men and cannot achieve significant upper body strength no matter how hard they try, women will get hurt and be unable to have babies if they train too hard . . ."

The purpose of this chapter is to explore modern research and educate women about their physical capacities. This chapter is not intended to argue whether or not a woman is capable of beating a man in a physical activity. I hope the male readers will take some time and enjoy this chapter. To the female readers, I say this: The responsibility for winning or making a lasting impression starts with you.

The argument against strength training

When talking about strength training, we mean *strength training*, not toning or losing fat, but becoming *physically* stronger. This requires that you work hard enough to develop hypertrophy (the growth of muscle). Common arguments made by women against strength training are that they fear losing flexibility, fear bulking up, or fear becoming unfeminine. These arguments are outdated, which I hope most women know by now. Besides, how could you *not* want a muscular body? A muscular body is attractive; it shows others that you take yourself and your art, sport, or training seriously. Besides, if building a muscular body were easy, there would be little need for a book like this, the average person would be winning bodybuilding competitions right and left, and you wouldn't see the same people spending hours at the gym every day.

A common argument made against women's strength training is that women just don't have the genetic capacity to develop strength to any reasonable degree. But the fact is that women are capable of doing as many full pushups, situps, even pull-ups as men, with proper training. Ladies, if you are to get anywhere with this, the first thing you need to do is rid yourself of old stereotypes and beliefs.

In his book, The Competitive Edge, published in 1980, Col. James L. Anderson of West Point Military Academy states: "West Point's fitness experience with men goes back over 150 years. Depth research of American women's fitness began four years prior to their admission to the Academy and has included the study and testing of several thousand women. In the beginning of this research we were attacked by two different camps: the Neanderthals, who thought women should literally stick to their knitting, and the active feminists, who insisted that women can do anything men can do and still have babies. We have tended to side with the feminists." This passage is especially interesting because West Point is a traditionally male only academy, and not until 1976 did women gain admission. It is only natural to think that West Point would tend to side with the Neanderthals, and not with the feminists, on the issue of women's strength and fitness. When I first read this back in the beginning of my martial arts career nearly 20 years ago, I felt that the author was way ahead of his time.

Gender difference

As far as strength training goes, the only real difference between men and women is the fact that we call ourselves men and women. In other words, women are not different to the point that it warrants special training or lower expectations. These are outdated notions that don't serve the female athlete. Women do not jeopardize their ability to have babies by doing physical work that requires lifting or a lot of upper body strength. The biggest hurdle women have to overcome is their own disbelief in their abilities. While it is wrong to automatically give men attributes such as muscular strength, it is also wrong to automatically give females attributes such as better flexibility. Many women appear more flexible than men because they are shorter and have shorter legs, thus they have a shorter distance to reach when bending over to touch their toes. Likewise, many men appear stronger than women, because they are bigger, taller, and have longer limbs. I will explain the importance of the length of the limbs in the next subsection. In addition, no woman should rely on general statistics, which are often based on the average values for sedentary people. Relying on general statistics or outdated notions provide lower expectations of women, and therefore don't give females the training they deserve and are capable of.

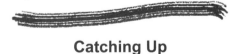

Catching Up

Because of outdated notions, many women have not participated in an adequate strength-training program, so they have a little farther to go to catch up with their male counterparts. This does not matter. What matters is that women do have the ability to catch up.

Female muscle tissue is identical to male muscle tissue; women just don't have the ability to grow their muscles to the same size (in general). Women can still reach substantial increases in muscular strength without a great deal of hypertrophy. Here are a few truths about female strength training:

• Since the muscle composition is the same in men and women, there is no need for women to engage in a special strength-training program designed just for women. Women and men can use the same types of training and the same types of exercises. Although male and female are different genders, strength training is not gender specific.

• Since muscle tissue is the same in men and women, the force exerted by equal size muscles is also the same in men and women. Men generally have larger muscles, but the individual muscle fibers in men do not have a greater ability to generate force than the individual muscle fibers in women.

• Women can handle the same intense sports conditioning as men and can perform on any level of competition, including the elite. Strength training for women is extremely beneficial and will not make you bulk up.

• Women, because they normally are not subjected to sports in the same way as men are, often need a little longer to catch up, mainly in terms of upper body and gripping strength. But when saying a little longer, we mean a *little* longer. Not years, but months.

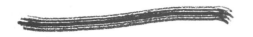

Gripping Strength

Wrist and hand strength is important in grabbing arts. Women generally have smaller hands than men, so if a woman is forced to grab the arm or wrist of a male opponent, she is at a disadvantage. If you reverse the scenario, it will be easier for a male, who has bigger hands, to secure a good grip around the smaller arm of a female. Good gripping strength is also important because it gives you a psychological advantage; it shows your opponent that you are serious about your attempt to control him.

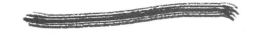

Absolute strength comparisons fail

When comparing male and female strength, we normally do so by comparing absolute strength; in other words, how many pounds you can lift once in a bench press. We don't take body size into consideration. A person who is smaller in size is generally also weaker in absolute strength. This is true regardless of whether the person is male or female. Thus a 200-pound woman will be stronger than a 100-pound man, and vice versa. When strength is evaluated in relation to body size, length of limbs, muscular size, and lean mass to fat ratio, there is no difference between male and female strength. Here is what I'm talking about:

To understand the male/female differences, you must place things in perspective. As an example, I have loaded bags, mail, and freight for Delta Air Lines for 20 years. Being a woman of relatively small stature (5'6" and 125 lbs) in this type of physically demanding job gave me an interesting insight one day, when one of my male peers said that I was the strongest person per pound he knew. The interesting concept here is "per pound." The old argument is that women are not as capable as men, and should therefore stay away from physically demanding jobs. But I could make another argument by saying that women actually work harder than men, and therefore deserve better pay for their efforts. In comparison to her bodyweight and height, at my job a woman must apply herself more in order to load an equal amount of cargo on an airplane as a man. And women do this every day. They load equal amounts of cargo in equal amount of time as their male peers. If a woman lifts more pounds per bodyweight than a man does, she is actually stronger. If a woman runs more steps than a man does in the same amount of time, she is actually faster. In other words, it is not as simple as making the observation that men have greater absolute strength than women (1-repetition deadlift, for example). You must also look at the factors that give you this perception.

Here is another example of how size, and even dress, affects a woman's apparent strength: Let's get back to my work with Delta Air Lines, loading baggage and cargo on the airplanes. If you are dressed too warm, you can't cool yourself efficiently and will have less apparent strength. Baggage handlers work outside and often in 100-degree summer temperatures. Since women wear bras, women are always hotter than men. If men don't believe this is enough to make a difference, wear a tank top under your regular shirt one day and compare. Because women are generally smaller than men, they must also lift the cargo higher in relation to their own height. While a man must lift only midsection high, a woman must lift chest high; while a man must lift chest high, a woman must lift above her head. At my job, women do this consistently, eight hours a day, five days a week, for 20 or 30 years! In short, men work under easier conditions than do women. During the course of the day, women demonstrate considerably more strength than do the male workers. So when I'm asked why I can't lift a 100-pound piece of cargo and place it on the top shelf, it is because I have to lift it above my head, and because it constitutes 80 percent of my bodyweight, and not 50 percent of my bodyweight. If the shelf were higher up, it is unlikely that a man would perform with the same kind of strength he demonstrated when he only had to lift hip or chest high.

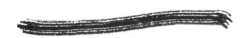

The Full Picture

If strength comparisons between men and women are to have meaning, they must be expressed and measured in relation to the surrounding conditions.

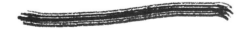

I found an interesting study regarding male and female athletes that kind of ties in with this: Research studies have shown that male quickness and superiority is due to their height and not their ability. For example, when running, "men are taller than women and therefore take longer strides." (Peak Performance Online, www.pponline.co.uk) When male and female athletes' performances were based on their heights, "the fastest woman in the world is almost 2 percent faster than the quickest man!" (Peak Performance Online, www.pponline.co.uk) Similar results have been found in swimming, which is an exercise that relies on good upper body strength. When taking the athletes' heights into consideration, in 1993, the female world champion, Jane Evans, was 2.5 percent faster than the male world champion, Vladimir Salnikov.

The next question is, how do women fare compared to men regarding muscle power? Again, if bodyweight and height are taken into consideration, studies have shown that women and men perform equally well, for example, in the vertical jump, which is generally used to measure leg-muscle power.

Let's look at muscular recovery after strenuous exercise next. You guessed it: "New scientific research suggests that females actually lose less strength than males during the course of a rigorous workout, and recover their muscular prowess more rapidly after an exhausting bout of exercise." (Peak Performance Online, www.pponline.co.uk) In a study done on male and female power-lifters in Finland, who performed 20 maximal squat lifts, it was found that, "muscles' ability to contract powerfully and quickly changed negatively by 28 percent in the males over the course of the workout, but dropped off by only 19 percent for females. Females also recovered from the 20-

lift session more quickly. One hour after the workout, female lifters' leg muscles could generate about 92 percent as much force as before the session, while male muscles were just 79 percent as strong. Finnish research suggests that quicker recoveries from truly taxing workouts are achieved by the fairer sex, even though coaches usually make killer workouts the exclusive domain of males."(Peak Performance Online, www.pponline.co.uk)

These studies support the idea that women are at least equal to men in strength as long as fair comparisons are made that take into account physical height and training background. Studies have also shown that males and females respond to training in a comparable manner. In other words, there is no need to think that women require some sort of specialized training solely based on the fact that they are female. In fact, this kind of thinking is destructive to the female athlete. I want to re-emphasize that the reason I bring this up is not to argue male vs. female abilities, or who is the stronger/ better athlete. There are too many factors outside of gender that influence a person's ability to make it to the top. This chapter is meant to be a motivational attempt to help women realize their true capacities. Ladies, do not go to your training half-heartedly, and never use the excuse that you can't do something because you are female! This simply isn't true, and you are pulling a lot of negativism on yourself and other women who are coming up through the ranks. If you are doing pushups on your knees, now is the time to get up on the balls of your feet and start training properly for the full pushup.

Conclusion

When evaluating differences between male and female, we must examine to what degree a particular strength has been used prior to the test. For example, if both men and women walk 5 miles a day, their legs will be equally strong relative to their body size. But if men also engage in weight lifting or a job that requires working the upper body while women sit at an office desk, male upper body strength is likely to be greater than female upper body strength relative to body size. In order to get a true test of male-female strength differences, the men and women tested must have trained under similar circumstances for similar periods of time, and the test must take into consideration physical build, such as body size and lengths of limbs. For example, if you are shorter than average, you will take smaller strides when running; if you are taller, you will take longer strides. The primary reason there is a difference in speed between people is because of different length legs, not because of different gender.

In the end, we tend to choose our sport because of our genetic potential. Just as a basketball player didn't grow tall as a result of playing basketball, a competitive female bodybuilder didn't develop large and highly defined muscles as a result of lifting weights. What, you say? Then why should she lift weights? Well, the fact is, she discovered that her genetic composition was favorable to developing large and defined muscles, and she chose bodybuilding because she felt this was a sport in which she could excel. The bottom line is that any person, man or woman, who lifts weights, will grow his or her muscles and develop strength. But only those with favorable genetics can compete in bodybuilding on the championship level.

Mental Approach to Strength Training

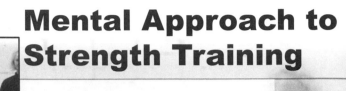

In this section:

- Mental readiness

- Strength and stress

- Winning attitude

- Setting a goal

- Genetics and mental drive

Mental Approach to Strength Training

So you have decided to get with the program and build the kind of strength that sets you apart from the pack. Having that winner's edge is important, even if you practice the arts for harmonious reasons and not for the ring or street. Winning enhances the human spirit; it makes you seek greater heights, makes you wonder where your limits are and if you can surpass them. Winning in a tournament is a temporary victory; winning over yourself is a lasting victory that leads to a feeling of exhilaration. But how do you get there?

Your physical training, skills, and attributes won't get you far if you don't have the will to succeed. Winning must matter to you; it must not only be more important than taking second place, it must be *significantly* more important. Start by defining what motivates you. Once you know this, training will mean more because it takes you a step closer to winning; it gives you self-mastery and makes you a tough competitor. When you start seeing the success your strength training brings you, you will find greater motivation to train even harder.

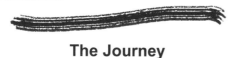

The Journey

A dedicated martial artist admires others who are skilled, strong, aggressive, quick, and intelligent. A dedicated martial artist studies these people and learns how to do better at his or her own game. This act of continuous improvement, of skill building and strength, gives you the motivation to do even better. This is why it is often said that the journey is more important than reaching the goal.

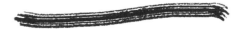

Mental readiness

Your mental approach to strength training affects your performance. When you can't be where you are, when your mind is not where your body is, you are unable to gain maximum benefit from any program. When tackling your strength goals, first clear your mind so that you can give your goals an all out effort. How do you clear your mind? First, make a commitment to strength training. You are training not only for today, but for the long haul. This means that you must prioritize your training over other duties. Once you approach your training with this commitment in mind, you will be more excited about going to the gym, your pain threshold will rise to where you can tolerate heavier weights and more repetitions, and you will realize greater muscular growth.

Let's take a minute and stir up some old ideas about martial arts training. We are often told to relax prior to a competition, test, workout, or sparring session. In real self-defense situations, too, we are told we will do much better if only we can relax. My question is: How do you relax when the combat arts, and especially a real threat on the street where your life is at stake, require a high degree of alertness? Is it possible that you might fare better if you take the opposite approach? Try this: Instead of doing relaxation exercises and meditation prior to an event, get a little worked up over it. Yes, come to the event physically and mentally prepared, but welcome the tenseness and the fear. It means you are ready. Relaxation exercises are good when done long before an event, or after the event, but not in the minutes preceding it. This is when you need to be fully alert, warmed up, and ready to go. Try the same concept when going to the gym to strength train: In order to properly alert your body, your mind should be on *it*, whether that is a contest, a demonstration, a belt promotion, a martial arts class or seminar, or simply a day at the gym.

Mental readiness is a prerequisite for physical readiness. Prior to going to the gym, rid yourself of mental baggage you might be carrying. If you can't do this, resolve your problems first, and then go to the gym. Once you step inside the doors, the gym is the only world that exists, and you should be ready to work.

Strength and stress

Stress is primarily a process of a sense of need to act on a set of demands. The nervous system is comprised of the brain and different types of nerves. Messages are sent from the brain through the nerves, and to the muscles and organs of the body. The autonomic nervous system conveys impulses from the blood vessels and all organs, the chest, abdomen, and pelvis through the nerves and to different parts of the brain. The autonomic nervous system is further broken down into two major components: the sympathetic and the parasympathetic nervous systems. The central part of the adrenal glands contains sympathetic nerve cells that react to excitement, fear, and stress. The events that are set off in our bodies as a result of this reaction are called stress responses, and take the form of turning off non-essential functions, such as blood supply to the gut and skin, the production of saliva (that's why your mouth gets dry when you're afraid or under stress), and certain brain functions such as ability to concentrate or think rationally. This prepares your body for meeting an emergency. The bad thing is that you also lose many of the martial arts skills you may have spent years to learn. Your fine motor skills and eye-hand coordination, such as your ability to apply a joint lock, intercept a strike, or wield a weapon with precision, may be lost in order to compensate for the need for gross motor skills, such as your ability to run away. As your heart rate quickens, your body begins to experience additional effects, such as tunnel vision, hearing loss, or memory loss.

When you are under stress to perform, years of experience might go out the door because your body becomes so focused on survival. In order to benefit from your long background experiences, you must at least alleviate the stress somewhat, or you will be just like an untrained person entering a fight. You see this in competition all the time. The strategy the fighters have worked so long and hard to achieve is gone the moment the bell sounds for the first round, and the fight becomes a sloppy blur of arms and legs, with the fighter throwing the most punches winning. But here is the thing: Throwing a lot of punches requires a lot of strength and muscular endurance. If you have participated in a disciplined strength program for some time, your strength and endurance will come to assist you when you are under stress to perform and are unable to rely on your many years of skill building.

Winning attitude

To keep this from becoming a bunch of mumbo-jumbo, let me state up front that if you want to win in martial arts, you must pay a price. Approach your training with the attitude that it matters and that you won't settle for anything but the best. This helps you establish a healthy mindset and good training habits. When you go to martial arts class or competition, your confidence will carry over to your performance. You will radiate an aura that communicates that you want to be exactly where you are, and nowhere else. As a result, others will feel your command presence and give you their attention. Never tell yourself that an exercise can't be done simply because you are older, female, smaller, or lack the genetic predisposition. You may not become the world champion in every exercise, but you can always go a step further than where you are right now. Train with the attitude that if your buddy (or opponent) can, then you can, too. When you discover what you are capable of, you will begin to hunger for more, for the opportunity to explore new frontiers of the human body and mind.

A good way to test how far you have come is through competition. Competition in any form, whether in a tournament with thousands of spectators or in silent competition within the training hall, serves to test your skill, strength, and endurance. Competition shows you the areas where you are weak. Going up against others who are stronger or better gives you the drive to seek out new avenues.

How you feel about winning or losing is also related to the number of people in the contest. If you take second place in the boxing ring, it has far different implications than if you enter a race with 10,000 competitors and take 50th place. But no matter how you look at it, it is far more satisfying to be up against people who are stronger and tougher than yourself and know that you have something to strive toward, than to already be the strongest and the best and wonder how you will find the drive to continue.

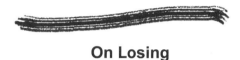

On Losing

Losing sucks! If you hate losing and being the weaker fighter, and most of us do, strength training will do a lot to help you achieve the image and physical edge you need to dominate your opponent in competition, on the street, or in silent comparisons in the training hall.

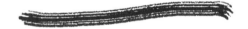

Remember this: When we talk about winning attitude, we are not talking about positive attitude. Just thinking that you can do something doesn't make you able to do it. It isn't quite that easy. If you're out of shape, no matter how positive your attitude is, you will not get in shape unless you pay the price in physical training time. But your mental attitude helps support your physical qualities, and vice versa. No matter how good a physical shape you are in, if you see yourself as defeated before the battle starts, you most likely are. To gain a mental edge on your opponent, you must have one basic ingredient: the will to gain an edge, the will to be better than he is. Pride in yourself and in your art helps you develop a competitive attitude. Pride doesn't mean arrogance; it means the ability to identify with the art, to become part of it to such an extent that when you practice it, it matters more than anything else. To rise above the rest and become truly good at your game, you must get involved not just physically, but mentally; your art must constantly be on your mind.

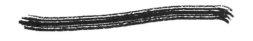

No Pain, No Gain

Yes, it is true! When training to become better or stronger, it is not necessarily whether you can beat your next opponent that should concern you, but rather how much pain you are willing to accept over how much pain your opponent is willing to accept. If you can take just a little bit more than him, you have started toward the road of accepting the pain of training as a necessary part of your regimen.

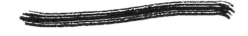

Setting a goal

When you go to the gym, train with the attitude of increasing strength and performance capabilities. For example, whether you run or swim for endurance, if you don't push it, you will not realize results. Whether you use weight machines or bodyweight exercises, if you don't push it, you will not realize results. How do you push it? You push it by not wasting time on socializing with other weight lifters. It also helps to have a goal; that is, a task goal and a time goal preferably written down, so that you know beforehand what you are

to accomplish and in what timeframe. Your written goal should state:

- What you want to accomplish
- The steps required
- How long it will take
- What you can expect to achieve

Listing your goal in concrete terms gives it meaning. If you leave out steps, you are likely to lose motivation somewhere along the way. You must also have some way of testing the benefits of your strength, or of comparing yourself to others so that you can see your advancement clearly. Consistency is important, but also specificity; that is, training that actually leads to strengthening the required body parts.

When setting your strength goal, it helps to know the requirements of your art. For example, your goal might be to pass the black belt test three months from now, which includes a physical strength requirement of 50 pushups, 50 situps, and a 3-mile run. Write it down. This is called your mission statement. In order for your mission statement to have meaning, it must:

- Make sense
- Be precise
- Be reasonable

In other words, "to pass the black belt test," might make sense and be reasonable if you have gone to class regularly, but since it lacks precision, it is a weak mission statement. Add the pushup, situp, and running requirement to give it precision and meaning.

Achieving your mission statement must contribute to a feeling of well-being. If it doesn't, you need to rephrase it, rethink it, or come up with a more reasonable mission.

In short, you must really want what your mission statement says. Next, keep track of your goal in writing, and mark off what you have done that advances you toward the goal.

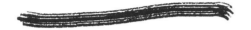

Mission Blooper

A mission statement that fails to identify the goal in precise and understandable terms is doomed to failure. For example, stating that you want to be the greatest in the world makes about as much (or little) sense as stating that you want to understand the meaning of life.

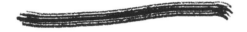

Oftentimes circumstances dictate the specific details of your goal. Prior to testing for my black belt in kickboxing, I set a training goal that included running, jumping rope, pushups, situps, and muscular endurance exercises. I decided on a reasonable schedule I could stick with and that would also help me improve my strength, endurance, and confidence. Then I wrote it down on a log-sheet, marking off every exercise I did for a period of three months prior to the test. If I missed a day or an exercise, I had to make it up within a week. Sometimes that meant an additional training session, and sometimes it meant just adding one or two exercises to a training session I was currently working on. After only a couple of weeks, I started feeling both stronger and prouder, which led to greater confidence on test day.

Many programs fail because they are too ambitious or complex, or because they completely lack a specific goal. A training log helps you measure how close you come to achieving your goal. It shows you where you were, where you are, and to where you are going. It is not enough to write down what you did, or even what you intend to do and whether you did it, you must also look ahead and know where you want to be two or three months from now. This might take some experimentation. Don't set goals that are too far out of reach. To stay motivated, you must see your progress and know that you can reach your goal as long as you follow the prescribed method and plan. If you are out of shape, try this for an upper body strength goal:

• Start with 5 pushups, and increase by 1 a week for 10 weeks, until you can do 15 full pushups with no cheating.

• If, after trying this for 2 weeks, it seems too easy, then increase by 2 pushups for 5 weeks instead of 1 pushup for 10 weeks, to reach your goal of 15 full pushups.

• When you have reached your goal, you can increase the number of pushups or change the type of pushup to make them harder. For example, try one-handed pushups and start back at 5, while increasing with 1 per week, until you are back at 15.

A continuous conditioning program requires a time commitment. Many people fail to make such a commitment and then cram in the weeks before the test or event. They feel they would rather put up with the pain of training for this isolated event, than put up with the pain of training all the time. This is a poor way of conditioning your body. If you see the martial arts as a life-long journey, you also need to engage in a strength and conditioning program that supports your martial arts training program. Having the technical skill but lacking the strength or endurance to use your skill is of little value.

Genetics and mental drive

We have discussed briefly how inherited physical traits contribute to success in sports. Our next question is: Is the winner's mindset inherent in our genes, or is it learned? Which influences winning more: your physical capacity or your mental capacity (mental edge, drive, desire to win)? Having both is ideal, of course, but many people have great physical capacity but lack the work ethics or the desire to participate in sports. These people's physical genetic inheritance will not help them win when they lack the mental drive to perform. Others have less than optimal physical capacity but have the work ethics and mental determination to succeed. Normally, these people will fare better. Without mental determination, you are not likely to get far. Much can be achieved when you will it to be achieved, regardless of whether or not you have good genes for physical activity.

In the beginning stages, good physical genetics that help you avoid appearing "clumsy" might be the more desirable attribute. But the mental edge becomes more important at the higher levels of training and competition. In the end, when you are physically ready, you are more likely to have emotional and psychological confidence and, therefore, be more mentally ready.

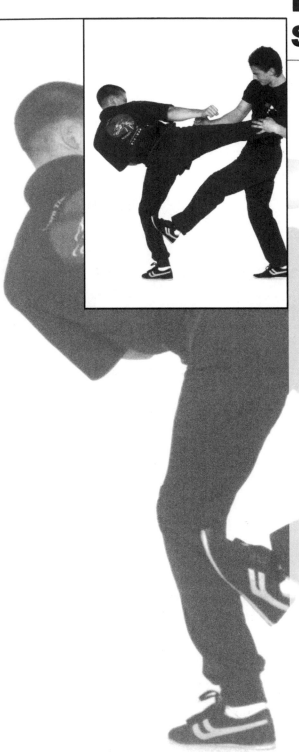

Introduction to Sport Specific Training

In this section:

- Benefits of sport specific training

- Types of sport specific strength

- Choosing your exercises

- Setting a training schedule

Introduction to Sport Specific Training

Are there specific strength exercises that will make you better at your particular martial art? For example, should a wrestler do different strength building exercises than a Tae-Kwon-Do practitioner? Should a kickboxer do different exercises than an Aikido practitioner? Keep the following in mind: Everybody's body functions in the same way. We all have the same sets of muscles, bones, and joints, and all our specific joint movements are identical. In general, exercises are therefore not sport or gender specific; we can all do the same types of exercises to strengthen the same types of muscle groups, regardless of who we are or what type of sport we are practicing. But although the exercises themselves aren't sport specific, the particular type of strength you need might be. For example, some sports require greater upper body strength than others. How you develop strength is general and equal for all people, but how you apply that strength in your sport or art is specific.

When designing a training program, you must also take injury prevention into account. For example, if your art requires you to take blows to the head, it is a good idea to develop strong neck muscles to reduce the likelihood of injury.

Now that you have built a general strength base and accumulated some knowledge about strength training, it is time to look at what you can do to acquire the type of strength your art specifically requires. But to do that, you must know where to start and how to continue through a progressive program. You are not to do this by trial and error. There is a better way.

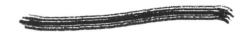

Strength Doesn't Always Look Like Strength

Strong neck muscles are essential in both the striking and grappling arts. Still, the neck is highly neglected in most strength training programs. One reason we tend to ignore strengthening the neck might be because neck strength normally doesn't show the way strong biceps or a washboard midsection show.

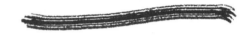

Benefits of sport specific training

A martial artist needs power, flexibility, endurance, agility, speed, and quick reflexes. All of these qualities are related to how strong your muscles are. For example, if you have muscular strength, you also have better speed and more power. But many people hate the conditioning routine because it is often painful or boring. In some ways, going to the gym might be how many of us felt about attending math class in high school: It was just an endless repetition of exercises that seemed to lead nowhere. In order to realize the value of any exercise (or math problem), you must see the benefits and know to where it leads. Training with sport specific skills in mind helps you see how your training benefits you directly in the performance of your art.

If you lift weights simply for the purpose of lifting weighs, you may not need to know anything about the strength requirements of a particular sport. But to the martial artist, this would be a waste of time.

Your goal is to enhance your martial art and make your muscular strength transfer to the art you are practicing. Remember, you must also avoid training in a way that alters your timing. This means that holding dumbbells or using ankle weights while punching or kicking is generally not a good idea.

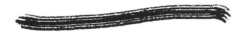

Strength for Skill Development

Strength training is not the skill itself; strength training is the mean that leads to better martial arts skills. If you want to improve specific skills, you must practice these specific skills. If you want to build strength for improving specific skills, you must develop stronger muscles. Don't confuse these two concepts.

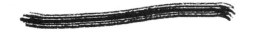

When analyzing the requirements of your art, many factors need to be examined and defined. Muscular strength relates to power, impact force, and mental superiority, and if improved performance is your goal, the quality of your training program is crucial. Remember that the purpose of strength training for the martial artist is to dominate your opponent through faster and more powerful and enduring movement. Think about how to achieve a complete approach to athletic performance. To gain a strength advantage, you must make an honest effort.

Training Tip

Most arts require movement that involves forceful trunk rotations; for example, throwing an opponent, or striking and kicking with power. Trunk twisting throws with a relatively heavy object, such as a sandbag weighing 30-50 pounds, can increase the rotational power of your trunk. Throwing lighter objects, such as a 12-pound medicine ball, does not have the same effect.

Types of sport specific strength

What are the demands of your sport? Not only what types of techniques does it require: punches, kicks, grappling, lateral movement, etc., but what particular demands do these techniques place on your body? A lot of lateral movement, for example, requires the ability to start and stop quickly, and may place stress on your ankles and knees. Does your art require mainly endurance? Are the moves performed during a longer period of time, such as in musical forms? Or does your art require mainly power and explosiveness, such as in board breaking? In order to determine what type of strength dominates in your art, look at those who are winning on the competition circuit and examine their qualities. Are they physically strong? Flexible? Fast? Here are a few examples of different types of strengths you might need in your art:

Balance Strength

The martial arts rely on balance and movement. For example, you might be fighting on uneven surfaces, on one leg (when kicking), or while being pushed or shoved. Training in exercises that use some instability help you develop the extra strength it takes to remain stable when in an unstable situation. For example:

• Lifting dumbbells is a more unstable exercise than lifting barbells, because one arm cannot assist the other.

• Doing abdominal work on an instability ball is a more unstable exercise than doing ab work on the floor.

• Doing situps with nobody supporting your feet requires greater control of your strength than if a partner is holding your feet steady.

• Doing pushups with one hand elevated develops differential strength between limbs and better control of your body.

Balance is an important element of power. If you lack balance, you lack power, no matter how strong your muscles are.

Starting Strength

The martial arts are dynamic, but they don't start that way. If you fight standing up, you will most likely start stationary and then initiate movement. If you fight on the ground, you will most likely start stationary from a stand-up position, initiate movement, and then go to the ground. If you are in a self-defense situation, you might be taken by surprise while you are standing, sitting, or lying down, or you might be in a position that requires a rapid start of movement in order to get away from your adversary. To begin movement, there must be an initial push against the ground. You must also have the ability to recognize a need to start movement, which involves reaction time.

• You can improve your ability to start movement by pausing in the middle of the concentric phase of a weight lifting routine. Then start the movement against the weight. As a variation, lie or sit down, and on a signal from your partner, get up and run across the room. The idea is to get from no motion to quick acceleration in the shortest amount of time.

• If your art involves a lot of starts and stops and changes in direction, train in short sprints with a lot of starts and stops. It helps if you have a partner who can motivate you and keep track of how fast you really sprint. It is easy to fall into the trap of running at a consistent pace. A sprint should be fast, followed by a short rest of perhaps a minute where you walk or do a slow jog, followed by another sprint.

Movement Strength

Most stand-up arts require both lateral and linear movement with quick changes in direction. In order to prepare for this kind of movement, you must practice this kind of movement. You don't improve in movement by practicing stationary exercises. Movement can include switching direction, going from standstill to full speed, from ground to standing, from standing to ground, and from standing to jumping. To be successful at movement, you must have enough strength in one leg to support your body through the change in direction. When training for movement, consider how much strength you have in a single leg.

• Single leg strength is required almost any time there is movement involved. The exception may be a jump that is initiated with both feet pushing off against the floor. Lunges and single leg squats help you develop single leg strength. Single leg squats can be done assisted at first, with your rear foot on a bench behind you. You can also start by sitting on a chair rocking forward and standing up, keeping one leg extended straight in front of you. If you need help moving your balance forward, hold dumbbells in your hands with your arms extended forward. Your weight should be toward your heel and not on the ball of your foot.

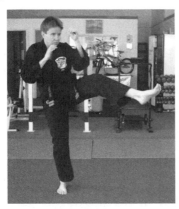

Single leg strength is important when throwing a kick, and anytime when moving with speed and explosiveness.

• Lateral movement speed is increased by pushing off with your rear foot, not by pulling forward with your lead foot. Do not lift your feet too high when shifting direction. Think of it as a quick shuffle. To move right, push with your left foot; to move left, push with your right foot. To move forward, push with your rear foot; to move back, push with your front foot. To avoid stressing your ankle or outside knife-edge, focus on landing toward the inside knife-edge or ball of the foot.

Kicking Strength

If your art is mainly a kicking art, you must find a way to strengthen the kicking muscles for more height and power in your kicks. The hip flexors are the main kicking muscles that enable you to lift your leg. If you can't lift your leg, you can't kick. The hip flexors are located at the front of the hip and lift the leg from the hip joint when you bring your thigh toward your abdomen, for example, when chambering your leg in preparation for a kick. Leg raises strengthen the hip flexors.

• Start by lying on your back and supporting your lower back with your hands.

• If you are strong enough to press the small of your back into the floor without arching your body, you can do leg raises with your hands behind your head.

• When this becomes easy, wear ankle weights or have your partner provide resistance to give you a better workout.

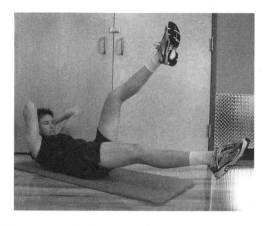

Mountain climbing is a good variation that can be done instead of leg raises. Hanging leg or knee raises are more difficult.

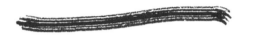

Training for Extra Weight

Most martial arts are practiced empty-handed, barefoot, and barefisted. But consider what happens when you put on sparring gear, wield a weapon, or add other weights that might be necessary in order to perform your art. How much energy does it drain from you? If you are using a weapon extensively, such as a sword or a staff, how can you train to build strength for wielding the weapon with power?

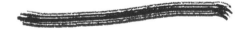

Choosing your exercises

Your goal is to improve your muscular system by doing the right kinds of exercises for the right time and duration, and to know when to expect a plateau and how to push past it without risking injury or impairment of your martial arts skills. Spending three hours a day at the gym, while working the machines and socializing with your peers, is not the most effective way to do this.

When choosing your exercises, know what you are striving to attain. Do you want to be able to lift a heavier opponent off of you in a grappling match and throw him onto the judges' table? Do you want to be able to outfight your opponent in a 10-round full-contact kickboxing competition? Do you want to persevere to the top in an 8-hour musical forms tournament for the Grand Championship with a movie offer tagged on? Different types of strength are required for each of these goals. In other words, training for the Grand Championship in musical forms does not necessarily prepare you for the grappling match.

When evaluating your sport specific strength and endurance, do so in an activity that simulates the requirements of your art. In other words, if you can run 10 miles, this is not necessarily an indication that you have the endurance to spar 10 rounds or to perform a demanding kata (form). One type of strength or endurance does not necessarily prepare you for another type of strength or endurance. Having the strength to bench press 200 pounds does not guarantee that you will have the strength to throw your opponent off of you in a grappling match, even if he weighs less than 200 pounds. Also consider the conditions under which the strength or endurance must be performed. Being able to spar or grapple for 30 minutes has little meaning, if you can't spar or grapple with enough speed or power or movement to outperform your opponent. Compare your current training regimen with your current condition. Then look at where you want to go and consider what changes need to be made.

• What type of strength is required? Is it quick muscular contractions (explosiveness)? Repetitive full-speed strikes? Lower body leg endurance?

• Will you be in constant motion, as in stand-up sparring, or will there be longer periods of time with little movement against great resistance, as in grappling?

• How much time is spent moving? What type of movement? Frequent starts and stops? Continuous movement? For how long do you need to maintain this particular movement?

• How long is a round of sparring? How many rounds do you spar? If you train for self-defense, how long is a realistic time for an altercation?

• How does your mobility, speed and power, explosiveness, and overall agility relate to the top players in your art? This should give you an indication of where you are and to where you need to go.

Next, determine the specific body parts you need to train in order to achieve greater strength or power for your particular martial art. Is it the legs? The trunk? The upper body? The arms? The neck? Why? If you can't answer these questions, you can't expect to design a program that will really work for you.

• If your art is Sumo, you probably need strong legs, a large body, and a stable base, more so than quick hands or feet. The same might apply to wrestling or any of the grappling arts.

• If your art requires you to clinch with your opponent and drive him into the ropes, you need strong legs.

• If your art requires you to score a quick point without being scored on, you need quick hands and legs, more so than overly developed legs.

• If your art requires wielding a traditional weapon, such as the nunchaku, staff, or sword, you need strong forearms and flexible wrists.

Setting a training schedule

Trying to peak in strength at a specific time is difficult for the martial artist, who practices his art all the time and never knows when he will have to use his skills for real. A specific training schedule designed to help you peak at a particular time is therefore not that useful. Rather, your program must be regular and disciplined. Training every day for a week, and then taking ten days off is not a regular or disciplined routine. You might feel disciplined when you train every day, but you are likely to run out of steam quickly and be unable to stick with such a program. In addition, the longer breaks in-between training sessions will defeat much of the progress you made. Once you get into a program, training every day might be an option depending on your mentality, but you must still research your training and be disciplined in order to reach results. Avoid getting into a rut. For example, training in short segments and with intensity is usually better than training for hours at a time.

A physical effort is required in order to accomplish your goal of getting stronger. It won't happen by reading a book or by trying the gym for two weeks without any specific plan or intention. How you plan your day is up to you and may depend on your work schedule and other obligations to home and family. But you should focus on using your time optimally. For example, you are not expected to spend four hours a day at the gym lifting weights in addition to your martial arts training at night. More does not directly relate to efficiency. Too much training can also affect your professional or home life negatively, or have other adverse effects, such as burnout. As a general rule: Try to limit the duration of your strength-training program to an hour each time. And, remember, you can achieve a whole lot in as little as 20 minutes. Intensity, specificity, and variety are more important than length of time.

Exactly how often or long you train is also determined by your specific goals. A younger martial artist, for example, might be training with the goal of winning several world titles, while an older martial artist might be training with the goal of practicing the martial arts for life without risking undue injuries. These programs require different approaches. Note that just because I used the younger and older martial artists as examples, it should not be assumed that these must be your goals, or that age in itself determines how you should train. What your goals are and how you tailor your training program are strictly individual matters.

If you decide to strength train on the same day you do your martial arts training, remember which has more importance. Strength training is designed to supplement and support you in your martial arts endeavors, not the other way around. Martial arts training should therefore take precedence. If possible, I recommend you do your martial arts training prior to your strength training to ensure that you are not too tired to go to class after a grueling strength workout. Your strength-training program should also be balanced with your martial arts training. I recommend two to three days a week in weight training in addition to your normal martial arts training of two to four days a week. If you have less time available, you can do a two-day a week program, but three days a week is recommended because it allows you to limit each session to an hour while still including all muscle groups each week.

You must do some experimentation to find the workout schedule that benefits you the most depending on your physical makeup, your time away for other obligations, and exactly what you wish to achieve in your sport. Just remember that when at the gym, work on what you had planned to work on, don't cheat, and don't stand around and talk. Improvements come as a result of a disciplined workout routine.

Training Tip

When designing a program, I recommend beginning with bodyweight exercises because they require no equipment, plus you condition yourself to getting used to moving your body as you must in your martial art. Also design a program with exercises that focus on many skills, such as balance and strength, and do exercises that work more than one muscle group at a time, for example, the squat instead of the leg extension. This makes the program more time economical.

Martial Art Specific Training Programs

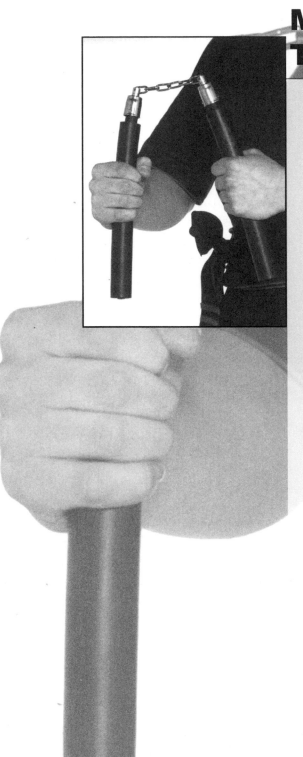

In this section:

Martial Art Specific Training Programs

Strength, in itself, does not give you better skills or guaranteed improved performance in the martial arts. But strength training helps you lay a sound foundation for improving performance; it gives you the potential to become better, stronger, faster, more dynamic, and more respected. The specific program you develop must consider the movements of your art, including start-stop, evasion, angling off, punching, kicking, throwing, falling, tackling, and wrestling techniques.

The program must be practical for building the type of strength that benefits you the most. Start by assessing your strengths and weaknesses and defining what your art requires. Your training can use many different concepts and exercises to meet these needs, but no two sports or martial arts require exactly the same athletic qualities. For example:

• If you are a well-conditioned stand-up fighter and you participate in a grappling session, you will undoubtedly feel sore the next morning because you have used muscles you normally don't use to that extent, and your body has been forced into positions you have not stretched or prepared for.

• If your art relies on explosive jump kicks, you might want to include a good dose of plyometric exercises to develop explosiveness. You also need a keen sense of balance and strong legs that allow you to jump.

• If your art includes sudden changes in direction, you must work on two areas: the particular muscles that help you change direction quickly, and the ability to move in the desired way. Sudden changes in direction require explosiveness, acceleration, and ability to start and stop quickly. Training in lateral movement exercises might be a good approach.

What to consider

We often stress the importance of upper and lower body strength equally, but if you have time constraints, it is more economical to consider what your art really requires and tailor your program accordingly. After all, your goal is to perform in your particular art, and not universally well in all types of sports. There are many ways you can design your program. The most limiting factor is the access to equipment. This does not mean that you limit your possibility to develop strength. For example, bodyweight exercises comprise some of the most efficient strength training exercises you can do. However, if you don't have access to a gym, you might limit the possibility of variety somewhat. When designing your program:

• Consider your current strength in your lower and upper body, and your current cardiovascular endurance. The drills you incorporate into your program must be possible to do at your current level, or you have to lower the requirements until you can do them.

• Consider where to train. Do you have access to a gym membership? Do you have weight-training equipment at home? If not, can you design a program that relies on just bodyweight exercises? Is there a track nearby where you can run?

• Consider what hours of the day you can train, and if you need a training partner in order to motivate you.

• Consider how vigorously you want to participate in your art. Do you train as a family activity, or do you compete frequently?

Next, to understand what type of strength you need in order to improve in your specific art, you need to do an analysis of what your art demands of your body. Does your art rely mainly on upper body, lower body, or cardiovascular strength? For example:

• How much upper body vs. lower body strength do you need?

• How much upper body vs. lower body flexibility do you need?

• How much movement or quick changes in direction does your art comprise?

• What types of speed are important: quick flicks of your hands, quick evasive moves and gap closures, or quick explosive moves against a heavier weight?

• How demanding is your art in cardiovascular terms?

• How many opportunities do you have to rest between matches, rounds, sets, or techniques?

When designing your program, strive for quality rather than quantity. Focus on what you are doing and toward what end it is leading you. If you spend hours at the gym or do 300 pushups a day, you will probably feel as though you are making great achievements initially, but you will also risk burnout real soon. Monitor how much stronger you actually become through your program. At what point do you feel you might have over-trained? If you have a day when you don't feel like training, ask yourself what brings about this feeling. Are you tired because you have trained too much? Is your body sore? Are you bored? Do you have little nagging injuries that seem to get worse with training? Your well-being should never be compromised as a result of training. Remember, your goal is to become a better, faster, stronger, and more respected fighter, and not a tired, hurt, or bored fighter.

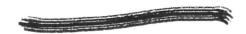

Time Off to Rest

Taking a complete week off to rest every three months or so is not going to hurt your strength and endurance; that is, if you feel like taking a week off. Taking time off to rest is not a requirement as long as you enjoy training.

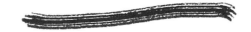

Designing your program

Now, let's move on to the specific training programs. Since there are so many styles of martial arts, as well as several eclectic styles that have emerged recently, I can only give you the main points of each "style-group." You can use this as a backbone for designing your training program, but any fine-tuning must be done after you have examined the details of the specific style you are practicing. You can find descriptions of the exercises in Chapters 6, 7, 9, 10, 11, and 12.

When choosing your particular routine, use the one listed for your art, or the one that most closely resembles your art as a guideline, and tweak it with the following in mind:

• Remember that you are training for martial arts, not for bodybuilding. You are training for functional strength, not for good looks.

• Set a program that you can live with for the long haul. Don't risk burnout or injury by being too ambitious early in the program.

• Work all of the muscles in your body with special focus on the muscle groups used the most.

• Work low repetitions, 2-3 sets and 6-10 reps, with relatively heavy weights. Rest approximately 2 minutes between sets.

• Work a variety of machines, free weights, and bodyweight exercises. If you have time for only one method, I recommend bodyweight exercises over machines or free weights.

• Do a few minutes of light stretching prior to and after your strength workout.

• You may substitute specific ab exercises listed in each program for the full abdominal workout described in Chapter 7.

• Remember that you still have to participate in martial arts training several times a week in addition to your strength training. Design your strength-training schedule to complement your martial arts schedule.

Karate

Many styles of martial arts fall under the blanket name "karate." When we say that we study karate, we generally mean that we study a stand-up type art that relies on both strikes and kicks as offensive weapons. The many styles of karate have different requirements, but since kicks are often thrown to the body and legs, great leg flexibility, although a plus, is not needed in order to succeed. Karate involves muscular strength in both the arms and the legs. For example, straight punches require powerful extension and retraction of the arm, backfists require strength in the shoulders, and front kicks require strong quadriceps and hip flexors. The karate practitioner needs:

- Balance through strong stances
- Ability to transfer strength from the legs to the arms through trunk rotations
- Ability to start and stop movement quickly when advancing and retreating

OPTION ONE	REPETITIONS
Leg Press (quadriceps)	8-8-8
Hamstring Curl (hamstrings)	8-8-8
Lying Leg Raise (hip flexors)	15-12-10
Bench Press (pectorals, deltoids)	8-8-8
Seated Row (latissimus dorsi, biceps)	8-8-8
Triceps Extension (triceps)	15-12-10
Medicine Ball Twist (obliques)	10-8-6 (alternating)
Sandbag Throw (abdominals, obliques)	10-8-6 (alternating)

Training Tip

Do the sandbag throw with a relatively heavy bag weighing 30-50 pounds. Throw the bag as far as you can while tightening your abs. Avoid over-extending your balance.

OPTION TWO	REPETITIONS
Squat (quadriceps)	15-12-10
Bench Step-Up (hamstrings)	10-8-6 (each side)
Hanging Leg Raise (hip flexors)	10-8-6
Pushup (pectorals, deltoids)	20-15-10
Inverted Row (upper back)	10-8-6
Chair Dip (triceps)	10-8-6
Diagonal Crunch (obliques)	15-12-10 (each side)
Reverse Crunch (lower abs)	15-12-8

Training Tip

If you need an easier version of the inverted row, place your feet on the floor instead of on a chair. The hanging leg raise is intended to strengthen the hip flexors, the main kicking muscle. If you need an easier version of this exercise, substitute hanging knee-ups.

Tae Kwon Do

Tae Kwon Do is one of the more popular martial arts in the United States. It, too, comes in a couple of versions with minor differences between schools. In general, Tae Kwon Do is a stand-up art that relies on both punches and kicks mainly from long range. Kicks seem to dominate, and many kicks are thrown high to the head. Board breaking is also practiced in many schools, so you need good hand and foot speed for the generation of power. The Tae Kwon Do practitioner needs:

- Balance, good single leg strength, and flexibility primarily in the legs
- Explosive footwork for quick in and out movement to score on an opponent while avoiding getting scored on
- Multiple kick endurance
- Explosive jump kick strength

OPTION ONE	REPETITIONS
Leg Extension (quadriceps)	8-8-8
Stability Ball Lift (glutes)	12-10-8
Bag Kicking (kick endurance)	3 X 1 minute
Bench Press (pectorals, deltoids)	8-8-8
Seated Row (latissimus dorsi, biceps)	8-8-8
Triceps Extension (triceps)	8-8-8 (each side)
Bent Leg Crunch (upper abs)	15-12-8
Reverse Crunch (lower abs)	15-12-8

Training Tip

Throw continuous mixed kicks during the heavy bag kicking exercise. Vary the routine by throwing only front kicks, roundhouse kicks, or sidekicks for one minute each. Rest for 30 seconds to a minute between rounds.

OPTION TWO	REPETITIONS
Jump Squat (explosiveness)	10-8-5
Power Skip (explosiveness)	10-8-5 (alternating)
One-Legged Squat (quadriceps)	6-4-2 (each side)
Shoulder Rotation (shoulders)	8-8-8 (each side)
Lateral Raise (deltoids, trapezius)	8-8-8
Chair Dip (triceps)	8-8-8
Situp (upper abs)	15-12-8
Leg Raise (lower abs)	15-12-8

Training Tip

Start with the lower body plyometric exercise. If you are unable to do the full set, decrease by 2, for example, do 8-6-3 instead of 10-8-5. Rest 2-3 minutes between each plyometric set.

Hapkido

Hapkido is primarily a stand-up art that relies on punches, kicks, joint control holds, and takedowns. Because of the varied nature of the art, several types of strength are needed in the legs, upper body, and hands. Since you will get thrown, you must also know how to fall properly without getting injured, and you need strength and endurance for getting back up repeatedly during training. The Hapkido practitioner needs:

- Good balance for kicks, takedowns, and throws
- Shoulder strength to avoid injury during joint locks, shoulder locks, and throws
- Gripping strength to execute locks with intent

OPTION ONE	REPETITIONS
Leg Press (quadriceps)	8-8-8
Leg Curl (hamstrings)	8-8-8
Barbell Squat (quadriceps, hamstrings)	8-8-8
Bench Press (pectorals, deltoids)	8-8-8
Seated Row (latissimus dorsi, biceps)	8-8-8
Wrist Curl (forearms, wrists)	15-12-10 (flexion/extension, each side)
Diagonal Crunch (obliques)	15-12-8
Reverse Crunch (lower abs)	15-12-8

Training Tip

The barbell squat adds instability to lower body training and also works the hamstrings. If you feel unsure of the amount of weight you can squat, have a spotter on standby to assist you.

OPTION TWO	REPETITIONS
Squat (quadriceps)	15-12-8
Bench Step-Up (hamstrings)	10-8-5 (each side)
Resistance Band Foot (shins, calves)	15-12-10 (flexion/extension, each side)
Shoulder Rotation (shoulders)	8-8-8 (each side)
Lateral Raise (deltoids, trapezius)	8-8-8
Wrist Rotation (forearms, wrists)	15-12-10 (each side)
Side V-Up (obliques)	15-12-8
Pelvic Thrust (lower abs)	15-12-8

Training Tip

Wrist curls and wrist rotations strengthen the forearms and hands, which are used when gripping or applying joint locks. Add a grip strengthening exercise for an extra edge.

Judo

Judo is the art of unbalancing and throwing an opponent without going down with him. A judo practitioner relies on tying up an opponent while standing, and quickly manipulating his or her balance with a forceful throw. Although judo relies on manipulating an opponent's center of gravity, strength is important for speed and to overcome a resisting opponent in throwing and pinning techniques. The judo practitioner needs:

- Explosive power and coordination
- Lower body strength, upper body strength, and wrist and gripping strength
- Shoulder strength to guard against injuries
- Balance and explosive speed in hip rotations
- Abdominal strength for forceful throws

OPTION ONE	REPETITIONS
Barbell Squat (quadriceps)	8-8-8
Stability Ball Lift (glutes)	12-10-8
Jump Squat (explosiveness)	10-8-5
Seated Press (deltoids, triceps)	8-8-8
Shoulder Rotation (shoulders)	8-8-8 (each side)
Wrist Curl (forearms)	12-10-8 (flexion/extension, each side)
Medicine Ball Pass (obliques)	10-8-6 (to partner)
Medicine Ball Throw (abdominals)	10-8-6 (for range)

> ### Training Tip
>
> Use any medium-heavy object of 10-20 pounds in lieu of the medicine ball. Throw for range, or far as possible.

OPTION TWO	REPETITIONS
Frog Hop/Squat (quadriceps, endurance)	20-15-10
Bridge (glutes)	3 X 30 seconds
Calf Raise (calves)	20-15-10 (each side)
Plyometric Pushup (explosiveness)	8-5-3
Nunchakus (forearms, grip)	3-2-1 minutes (each side)
Crushing Grip Strength (forearms, grip)	15-12-8 (each side)
Stability Ball Crunch (upper abs)	20-15-10
Leg Raise (lower abs)	12-10-8

> ### Training Tip
>
> Do the frog hop/squat variation by holding the squat for 30 seconds between each set. Do the plyometric pushup with or without a handclap. Push up forcefully to allow your hands to leave the floor. Swing a baseball bat in lieu of the nunchakus.

Jiu-Jitsu

Jiu-jitsu is a grappling art that relies on quick takedowns, joint locks, and chokes mainly on the ground. The Jiu-jitsu practitioner normally starts standing up and executes a quick shoot at his opponent's legs to take him down. Joint locks require good gripping strength and leverage. Since much of the fight takes place on the ground, good leg strength is needed to move while sitting or kneeling, and to defend and counter an opponent's techniques. The Jiu-jitsu practitioner needs:

- Quick starting speed and explosiveness when shooting in for a takedown
- Balance for executing joint locks and takedowns with leverage
- Good gripping strength and strong upper arms for locking, grappling, and restraining techniques
- Neck strength to guard against injuries during neck control techniques and chokes
- Flexible feet for protection against foot and ankle locks

OPTION ONE	REPETITIONS
Leg Press (quadriceps)	8-8-8
Hip Adductors (machine)	8-8-8
Resistance Band Foot (shins, calves)	15-12-10 (flexion/extension, each side)
Incline Barbell Curl (biceps)	8-8-8
Parallel Bar Dips (triceps)	8-8-8
Crushing Grip Strength (forearms, hands)	15-12-8 (each side)
Weighted Neck Flexion (neck)	15-12-10 (straight and lateral)
Medicine Ball Situp and Throw (abs)	15-12-8
Good Morning (lower back)	8-8-8

Training Tip

The good morning is a lower back exercise. Start with a very lightweight bar, such as a bo-staff across your shoulders before increasing the weight. Do each move with good control to avoid hurting your lower back.

OPTION TWO	REPETITIONS
Frog Hop/Squat (quadriceps, endurance)	20-15-10
Hip Adductors (resistance band)	15-12-10 (each side, alternating)
8-Move Foot Exercise (foot and ankle)	5 of each move (each side)
Plyometric Pushup (explosiveness)	10-8-6
Triceps Pushup (triceps)	15-12-10
Newspaper Ball (forearms, hands)	2 times (each hand)
Neck Nod and Head Roll (neck)	15 (each direction)
Stability Ball Situp (abdominals)	12-10-8
Back Extension (lower back)	12-10-8

Aikido

Aikido is a defensive art that relies on circular moves to redirect an opponent's energy and use it against him, often to effect a throw. Much time is also spent kneeling and moving on the ground. When practicing Aikido, one person acts as the aggressor and the other as the defender. This means that if you are the aggressor you will get thrown a lot, so you need strength to get up from the ground repeatedly. Wristlocks and joint control techniques are used, so gripping strength is essential. Akido also uses traditional weapons, mainly the bo (long staff), jo (short staff), and bokken (wooden sword). The Aikido practitioner needs:

- Endurance for continuous repetition of exercises
- Balance and a strong midsection for doing pivots with power
- Shoulder strength to avoid injury when falling and during joint lock practice
- Wrist and forearm strength for wielding weapons with power
- Leg strength for kneeling and getting up from the ground

OPTION ONE	REPETITIONS
Leg Press (quadriceps)	8-8-8
Stability Ball Lift (glutes)	12-10-8
Jump Squat (explosiveness)	10-8-5
Lateral Raise (deltoids, trapezius)	8-8-8
Wrist Curl (forearms)	12-10-8 (flexion/extension, each side)
Wrist Rotation (forearms)	12-10-8 (each side)
Medicine Ball Situp and Throw (abs)	15-12-8
Trunk Rotations (obliques)	8-8-8 (each side)

Training Tip

The jump squat develops lower body strength and explosiveness as needed for getting up from the ground quickly. The jump squat, along with frog hops (included in option two), helps develop strength and ability to fight while kneeling and moving on the ground.

OPTION TWO	REPETITIONS
Frog Hop/Squat (quadriceps, endurance)	20-15-10
Bridge (glutes)	3 X 30 seconds
Calf Raise (calves)	20-15-10 (each side)
Shoulder Rotation (shoulders)	8-8-8 (each side)
Nunchakus (forearms, grip)	3-2-1 minutes (each side)
Crushing Grip Strength (forearms, grip)	15-12-8 (each side)
Diagonal Crunch (obliques)	15-10-8 (each side)
Sitting Knee Crunch (upper abs)	15-10-8

Training Tip

Good forearm strength is developed by swinging a weighted object. Since nunchakus are normally not part of Aikido training, you may substitute a bo-staff, jo-staff, or bokken.

Muay Thai/Kickboxing

Muay Thai and kickboxing are tough full contact arts that require considerable body conditioning. Both punches and kicks are thrown, and many kicks are thrown low impacting with the shin. Strong shins are therefore essential. Matches are fought in rounds similar to boxing, so you need the endurance to go the full round. Jumping rope is a great cardiovascular endurance builder. So are heavy bag work and mitt work. Bodyweight exercises, such as pushups, pull-ups, and squats help you establish the strength and competitive mindset needed to defeat your adversary. Since the art does not rely on a one-strike knockout (although one can hope for that), you need to be strong enough to outlast your opponent. A good Muay Thai/kickboxing training program is comprised of jump rope, frog hops, stair climbing, pushups, situps, pull-ups, heavy bag punching and kicking, and running. The Muay Thai/kickboxing practitioner needs:

- Upper and lower body strength
- Midsection strength for throwing powerful strikes and taking full power blows
- Neck strength to guard against whiplash injuries as a result of taking strikes to the head
- Muscular endurance to keep punching and kicking for the full length of the round

OPTION ONE	REPETITIONS
Leg Extension (quadriceps)	8-8-8
Resistance Band Foot (shins, calves)	15-12-10 (flexion/extension, each side)
Jump Rope (calves, endurance)	3 X 2 minutes
Decline Press (pectorals, deltoids)	8-8-8
Upright Row (upper back)	8-8-8
Pulldown (trapezius, latissimus dorsi)	8-8-8
Weighted Neck Flexion (neck)	15-12-10 (straight and lateral)
Medicine Ball Twist (obliques)	10-8-6 (alternating)
Sandbag Throw (abdominals, obliques)	10-8-6 (alternating)

Training Tip

The quadriceps and shins should be well-developed because the Muay Thai/kickboxer takes a lot of kicks to these areas. Foot flexion/extension exercises help develop the shins. Also try steep uphill hiking.

OPTION TWO	REPETITIONS
Frog Hop/Squat (quadriceps, endurance)	20-15-10
Toes Over the Edge Raise (shins)	15-12-10 (each side, alternating)
Running/Sprinting (endurance)	2-mile run (varied with sprints)
Plyometric Pushup (explosiveness)	10-8-6
Inverted Row (upper back)	8-8-8
Chin-Up (trapezius, latissimus dorsi)	8-6-4
Neck Nod and Head Roll (neck)	15 (each direction)
Situp (upper abs)	15-12-10
Side V-Up (obliques)	12-10-8 (each side)

Training Tip

Muay Thai/kickboxing are full contact arts where a knockout often wins the fight. Strong neck muscles are therefore crucial. Reserve time for training the neck in every session. Wind, or the ability to pick up the pace without running out of steam, is also crucial and can be developed through running mixed with sprint exercises. The chin-up (palms turned toward you) is a slightly easier version of the pull-up and can be done assisted if you lack good upper body strength.

Mixed Martial Arts

The mixed martial arts have become exceedingly popular during the last decade, after the advent of the Ultimate Fighting Championships. Mixed martial arts are demanding and include stand-up fighting and grappling, often in the same bout. Although many mixed martial arts competitions have time limits, some don't, and the bout goes on until one fighter is unable to continue. The mixed martial arts practitioner must be able to start standing up, quickly shoot at his opponent's legs and go for a takedown, and attempt to subdue his opponent on the ground. The mixed martial arts practitioner needs:

- Superior strength and endurance, physical size is helpful
- Explosive lower and upper body strength for shoots and grappling
- Good gripping strength
- Hand and forearm strength
- Neck strength to guard against injuries during neck control techniques & chokes

OPTION ONE	REPETITIONS
Jump Squat (explosiveness)	10-8-5
Barbell Squat (quadriceps)	8-8-8
Stiff-Legged Deadlift (hamstrings)	8-8-8
Bench Press (pectorals, deltoids)	8-8-8
Upright Row (upper back)	8-8-8
Crushing Grip Strength (forearms, hands)	15-12-8 (each side)
Weighted Neck Flexion (neck)	15-12-10 (straight and lateral, each side)
Incline Weighted Situp (upper abs)	15-12-8
Medicine Ball Throw (abdominals)	12-10-8

Training Tip

Increase the difficulty of the ab exercises by holding weights, or by doing them on an incline, head down. The steeper the incline, the more difficult the exercise is. Although it is necessary to stabilize your feet when doing incline situps, avoid pulling with your legs.

OPTION TWO	REPETITIONS
Frog Hop/Squat (quadriceps, endurance)	20-15-10
Side Lunge (quadriceps, glutes)	15-12-10 (each side, alternating)
Single Leg Curl (hamstrings)	15-12-10 (each side)
Plyometric Pushup (explosiveness)	10-8-6
Pull-Up (trapezius, latissimus dorsi)	8-6-4
Towel Twist (forearms, hands)	3 times (each direction)
Neck Nod and Head Roll (neck)	15 (each direction)
Stability Ball Crunch (abdominals)	12-10-8
Sandbag Throw (abdominals, obliques)	12-10-8

My Training Program

As of the writing of this book, I am 41 years old and have practiced the martial arts for 18 years. I practice three arts: Kenpo karate, kickboxing, and street freestyle, which includes punching, kicking, throwing, grappling, and weapons. I will now share with you a typical strength workout I do three times a week, which has given me the muscular strength, endurance, and confidence to outlast most opponents. Each session takes about an hour to complete and includes cardio training, lower and upper body endurance and strength training, and midsection exercises. I vary my routine about every three weeks, and sometimes I use two slightly different routines on alternate days. I include a lot of pushups. I also swim for endurance, cardio fitness, and total body conditioning for about forty minutes once a week.

All weight lifting is done with enough resistance to limit the repetitions to 8 per set and with no break between running and pushup segments, pull-up and pushup segments, or weight lifting and pushup segments. The midsection exercise is done without breaks until you get to the stretching segment.

If you want to try this workout, adjust it to your current fitness level. For example, do just 5 pushups instead of 20 between segments, start with assisted pull-ups instead of full bodyweight pull-ups, take a 1-minute break between exercises, or run at a slower pace. But remember, in order to get useful results, you must increase the difficulty of the training periodically. It doesn't take years to build good strength. A few weeks are enough to begin realizing results. No pain, no gain. Yes, it's true. GOOD LUCK!

Uphill Run Slight Incline (treadmill)

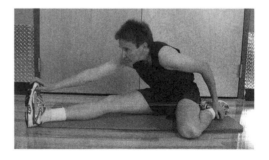

2 minutes stretching
2 minutes warm-up walk
3 minutes slow jog, 12 min/mile pace
20 pushups

2 minutes slow jog, 12 min/mile pace
3 minutes slow run, 10 min/mile pace
20 pushups

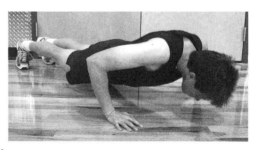

2 minutes slow run, 10 min/mile pace
3 minutes medium run, 9 min/mile pace
20 pushups

2 minutes medium run, 9 min/mile pace
3 minutes fast run, 8 min/mile pace
5 minutes cool-down, slow jog to fast walk
2 minutes stretching
50 pushups

Steep Uphill Climb (mountain climber machine)

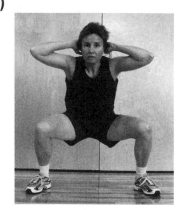

10 minutes, highest resistance and incline
10 bodyweight squats
50 pushups

Lower Body

Leg press, 3 X 8 reps
10 bodyweight squats
Hamstring curl, 3 X 8 reps
10 bodyweight squats
2 minutes stretching

Bodyweight Pull-Up Pyramid

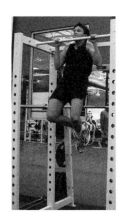

8 pull-ups, wide grip palms forward
10 hands wide pushups
6 pull-ups, wide grip palms forward
10 hands wide pushups
4 pull-ups, wide grip palms forward
10 hands wide pushups
5 pull-ups, lateral grip palms in
10 hands wide pushups
5 pull-ups, narrow grip palms rearward
10 hands wide pushups
5 pull-ups, wide grip palms forward
10 hands wide pushups

Upper Body

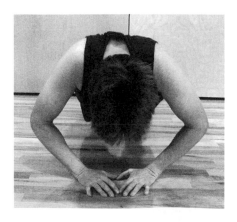

Seated row, 1 X 8 reps
15 pushups
Seated row, 1 X 8 reps
15 pushups
Seated row, 1 X 8 reps
15 pushups
Triceps extensions, 1 X 8 reps
10 hands narrow pushups
Triceps extensions, 1 X 8 reps

10 hands narrow pushups
Triceps extensions, 1 X 8 reps
10 hands narrow pushups

Midsection

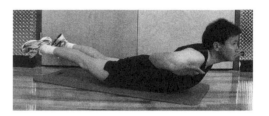

Mountain climbing, 20 reps each leg
Leg spread, 10 reps
Leg raise, 10 reps
Reverse crunch, 10 reps
Diagonal crunch, 10 reps each side
Side bend, 10 reps each side
Side V-up, 15 reps each side
Alternating reverse crunch, 15 reps
Crunches, 20 reps
Alternating diagonal crunch legs vertical, 15 reps each side
Straight crunch legs vertical, 10 reps
Sitting knee crunch, 15 reps
2 minutes stretching
2 minutes back extensions
20 pushups

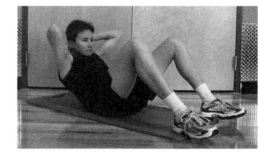

Conclusion

Everybody wants to know the secret. In my many years as a student and teacher of the martial arts, I have finally learned what it is: The secret is that there is no secret; there is only hard work. However, if I were forced to explain the secret in greater detail, I would say that strength wins.

There are so many ways you can be strong — physically, mentally, emotionally. An old friend once told me: "If it ain't right at home, it ain't right at work, either." By that he meant that you must keep your house clean and free of excess baggage in order to keep your mind clear and focused. Most of us probably remember Maslow's Pyramid of Needs from psychology class. At the base of the pyramid is survival, our basic need for food and shelter. Before this need is met, we cannot satisfy our higher needs of knowledge and self-actualization. In practical terms, this means that when you are hungry, tired, sick, overloaded with work, or weak from an argument with your spouse, you must clean your house first and take care of your basic needs before embarking on a higher journey. Once you have done so, your mind will be clear to focus on building strength and bettering yourself as a martial artist.

Strength is only valuable if it helps you achieve your goals. There is no quick fix to increasing functional strength (the type of strength used in your art). First, you must have knowledge of what is required. Then, you must put forth the effort to design a program. And, finally, you must have the dedication and work ethics to follow the program. Many of us complain that we are not "getting anywhere." But a common problem is that we don't do anything to push beyond our current condition. Yes, you must challenge yourself regularly. As you get stronger, you must push forward again. The principle of progressive overload teaches you that your efforts are never enough; that you will never arrive. I suppose this knowledge can be discouraging. But it does not need to take years to increase your strength. A good program and a conscious effort allow you to see definite results in just a few weeks.

Modern strength/weight training surpasses traditional methods, such as standing in the horse stance for an hour five days a week. But strength training is still a long-term project. Taking small steps allows your body to adapt and decreases the risk of injury while increasing motivation. Taking small steps allows you to educate yourself on your body. For example, if you get an annoying pain, a small adjustment in technique is often enough to ward off further injury. If you notice growth in the muscle group you are training, a small tweak of your technique might allow you to realize even greater growth. Progression is important, because your body isn't capable of performing a 10-mile run or 200 squats on the first day.

Don't continue in the same aerobic class year after year. It is not "toning" you want, but functional and impressive strength that helps you make use of the martial art secret. Remember, somebody else's program is not your program. Train with intent. Train with intent to explore more than what you find in this book.

About the Author

Martina Sprague has studied and taught the martial arts for eighteen years and has black belts in Kenpo karate, kickboxing, and street freestyle. She is a scholar of sports science, history, and warfare and has written several books on the martial arts, in addition to two books on Scandinavian and Viking war history. You can reach Martina via her website: www.modernfighter.com.

Index

U

upper abs 112, 162–163
upper back 143–145
upper torso 37
upright row 143

V

variation 83–84

W

warm-up 118, 124, 185
weapons 23, 27, 68
weighted neck flexion 152–153
weight loss 176
wrist curl 149
wrist rotation 150

Also Available from Turtle Press:

Timing for Martial Arts
Complete Kickboxing
Ultimate Flexibility
Boxing: A 12 Week Course
The Fighter's Body: An Owner's Manual
The Science of Takedowns, Throws and Grappling for Self-defense
Fighting Science
Martial Arts Instructor's Desk Reference
Guide to Martial Arts Injury Care and Prevention
Solo Training
Solo Training 2
Fighter's Fact Book
Conceptual Self-defense
Martial Arts After 40
Warrior Speed
The Martial Arts Training Diary
The Martial Arts Training Diary for Kids
TeachingMartial Arts
Combat Strategy
The Art of Harmony
Total MindBody Training
1,001 Ways to Motivate Yourself and Others
Ultimate Fitness through Martial Arts
A Part of the Ribbon: A Time Travel Adventure
Herding the Ox
Neng Da: Super Punches
Taekwondo Kyorugi: Olympic Style Sparring
Strike Like Lightning: Meditations on Nature

For more information:
Turtle Press
PO Box 290206
Wethersfield CT 06129-206
1-800-77-TURTL
e-mail: sales@turtlepress.com

http://www.turtlepress.com